Happy & Healthy

A Wellness Journal of Baby's First Year

Peter L. Richel, MD, FAAP

LYONS PRESS
Guilford, Connecticut
An imprint of Globe Pequot Press

To buy books in quantity for corporate use
or incentives, call **(800) 962-0973**
or e-mail **premiums@GlobePequot.com.**

Lyons Press is an imprint of Globe Pequot Press.

Editorial Director: Cynthia Hughes Cullen
Editor: Lara Asher
Project Editor: Tracee Williams
Text Design: Diana Nuhn
Layout: Nancy Freeborn

Library of Congress Cataloging-in-Publication Data is available on file.

ISBN 978-0-7627-7376-3

Printed in the United States of America

10 9 8 7 6 5 4 3 2 1

The health information expressed in this book is based solely on the personal experience of the author and is not intended as a medical manual. The information should not be used for diagnosis or treatment, or as a substitute for professional medical care.

For my wife, my daughters, and my mother . . .

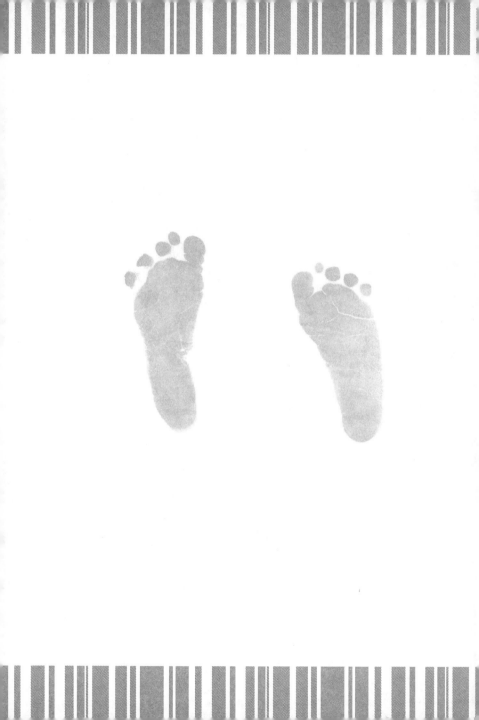

CONTENTS

ACKNOWLEDGMENTS

*I thank God for His Grace and for all of the blessings
He has given to me . . .*

My wife Sandy, for her endless love and support.

My daughters Lauren and Leanna, for teaching me how to be a father.

My mother Amy Bullett Richel, for giving me her love of children.

My pediatrician and mentor Dr. Arnold Tanis, for showing me the way.

My senior resident, Dr. Marilyn Caramore, for teaching me the way.

My 36 Smith family, for their dedication to all of our patients.

*My colleagues, Drs. Susan Liebeskind, Elizabeth Virginia-Hartman,
Vicky Zouzias, Sona Mehra, Lauren Budow, and especially
my partner Dr. Nick Germanakos.*

*My hospital, Northern Westchester Hospital, for their dedication to medical
excellence and compassionate patient-centered care.*

My musical partner, Gary Fry, for bringing my words to life.

*My friends, Cynthia Hughes, Lara Asher, and Tracee Williams for
being the coolest ladies in the publishing world.*

My patients, for keeping me smiling and singing every day.

I am forever grateful for each of these blessings . . .

INTRODUCTION

Preparing for Your Newborn

Congratulations! You are expecting a baby, and by now perhaps you are growing, showing, and glowing. Pregnant women truly radiate. It is lovely and attractive, so relish your appearance as your body changes. Remember this as you deal with the physical and emotional changes that every pregnant gal endures. As you know, you will gain a bit of weight and change shape temporarily, but it will all be worthwhile on your day of delivery.

It is so important that you maintain good health in general so that the growing fetus remains healthy as well. Routine visits to your obstetrician are necessary, and following his or her guidance is imperative. Your doctor and his or her staff will provide you with prenatal vitamins and advice regarding a well-balanced dietary intake. You will also undergo routine lab work and ultrasound surveillance during your pregnancy. This prenatal care is vital to the health of your baby. Regular exercise is also a must, so that you will be prepared for the delivery itself, and so that you will spring back to shape in the days, weeks, and months following delivery. Exercise can be passive, as with yoga, or it can be active, as with jogging.

Your emotional health is just as important as your physical health and well-being. Your partner or significant other is your best support and greatest advocate. He or she is the one who will be in your corner from start to finish. If you are a single mom, please be certain to ask a trusted friend or family member to join you on this journey. It is best to keep your partnership close during these months, for you will be better prepared, and even less likely to suffer from postpartum blues. So enjoy this time in your life . . . you are so special!

Obstetrical Visits

Regular visits with your obstetrician should be scheduled in advance with the same doctor for good continuity of care. Prenatal vitamins are a must as a dietary supplement for your health and for the health of the growing fetus. Routine lab work will be advised during the pregnancy to monitor your status from within.

Serial ultrasound evaluations will be ordered as a standard of care to observe your baby's growth over time during fetal life.

Nutrition

A well-balanced dietary intake is necessary, both for yourself and for your baby. A healthy weight gain is twenty-five to thirty-five pounds. Remember all of the food groups as you plan meals; refer to www.mypyramid.gov. Vegetarians may continue their diet, but be certain to take in enough protein, and supplement vitamin D, iron, and vitamin B12. Water is essential for you to maintain good hydration. This means drinking and tinkling all day long!

Stretch and Grow

Regular exercise should begin before you become pregnant. If not, start right away! You need to be in shape for labor and delivery. Everything in moderation . . . begin slowly and make thirty minutes a day your goal. Swimming and walking are both wonderful ways to stay in shape for delivery and beyond. Stretching is vital as well, and can be accomplished with yoga routines.

Regular exercise will improve your level of energy, increase your strength, and prepare your body for delivery.

Preparing Daddy

You are in this together—two is company; three is a family. You are embarking on an incredible journey, and you are doing it together. Real men admit that this can only be accomplished by a woman. Men may be able to play nose tackle in the NFL, but they should readily admit that they could never bear a child. This means that you deserve all of his love and support and partnership throughout the process of pregnancy.

In addition to being supportive of you, he must prepare for parenthood as well. He should take some time to do his own reading about how

MAKE A DATE WITH YOUR MATE!

There is no substitute for the bond that you share, beginning with your courtship, continuing through your engagement and marriage, and now through the dawn of expanding your family with your baby. Be certain to make time for each other, despite busy work schedules. You can read together, shop together, exercise together, attend classes together, or just relax with each other in the comfort of your home. Consider an outing to shop for baby needs—items that you have not received from friends and loved ones as gifts or at baby showers. If you have a meal out at the same time, all the better to spend that quality time together planning and discussing the future. It's wonderful to have him with you at prenatal classes and at your obstetrical visits if possible. This ensures that you will both be on the same page throughout your pregnancy. Stay close and connected, now and forever!

to care for a newborn. Ask your obstetrician about the availability of prenatal classes, usually offered by his or her office or at your local hospital. Bring your man along! Also, avail yourselves of a tour of the labor and delivery suite at the hospital at which you will be delivering the baby. This is informative and will allow you both to feel that much more comfortable when it is time for you to be admitted.

The role of the expectant dad goes beyond childproofing your home, painting the nursery, and setting up the crib. It is imperative for him to be your go-to guy for support on any level. He must prepare himself for parenthood and hold your hand from start to finish. He should also be emotionally well in order to support you now, during labor and delivery, and once the family arrives home.

Being in good physical shape is important for both of you, as nights can be long in the first weeks of your baby's life with you. Get him to exercise with you!

Take a Tour

Most hospitals offer prenatal classes for expectant parents to attend, with little or no fee. These are really valuable. At these classes you can learn about the most current recommendations for breast-feeding, bottle-feeding, circumcision, and more. In association with a prenatal class, tours of the labor and delivery suite are often offered as well. Take advantage of a tour, and the surroundings will not seem foreign to you when you are admitted. Doing these things with your partner is fun, informative, and time well spent. In fact, it is invaluable!!

Go Shopping

Go on a shopping spree together! Whether it's an item for the nursery, a special soft toy for baby, or adorable little outfits, making these purchases as a team will give you special parent bonding time. Enlist him in the choices. Try not to micromanage the list or the purchases under the guise of "moms know best." Active involvement in shopping for your baby's needs will keep him interested and invested in the process, and he will feel wanted and needed.

Preparing Your Home

Is your home ready to receive your most precious possession? Now that you are both preparing for your baby, we must consider adapting your home. Whether you live in a house, a condominium, or an apartment, you are expanding the family, and that takes some deliberate planning. The most important consideration is safety. Remember, it's never too early to start childproofing the home, even though it will be many months before your baby will actually be able to investigate his or her surroundings and find potential danger. That means it's time to go shopping!

After the fun task of purchasing a crib and/or bassinette, a changing table, a high chair, and all of the necessary baby products available today, it is prudent to be armed with items such as electrical plug covers, safety latches for doors and cupboards, and carbon monoxide monitors. We are waging a war against danger! Look for baby gates as well, particularly if you will need to protect your crawling infant from any stairs. Toxic products should be elevated to a height that is well out of reach. You might even consider purchasing thin carpet pads to place beneath small carpets so that they won't slip under your feet as you walk with your baby. Later on, when he is toddling, those rugs will be stable for him as well.

If you are doing any construction in preparation for the homecoming, it's best to accomplish it well in advance of the birth. Ideally, the nursery should be clear of any construction dust or fresh paint fumes weeks prior to baby's arrival. Dust and fumes are irritants that can be harmful to a newborn's airways. Always err on the side of caution when considering how to best prepare the home for your new baby. Preventive medicine is the best medicine!

Important Health Items

Babyproofing means making your home danger proof for infants. Medicines and toxic chemicals (cleaning supplies) must be well out of reach or in securely locked cabinets. Lead-based paint may have been used in homes built prior to 1978. This paint should be tested, as exposure and subsequent increased lead levels in infants and children can affect their physical health and their development.

A Crib in Your Crib

Be sure that your baby's crib meets certain requirements. Sides need to be lockable. The slats should be no greater than 2⅜ inches apart; this is important because the baby's head must not be able to go through and become lodged. The crib mattress should be firm and fit snugly.

If you are using a hand-me-down or vintage crib, be sure that lead paint is not an issue, as this can be toxic to the infant, especially later in her first year of life when she pulls to stand and gnaws on the crib rail.

Way Down Low

Imagine yourself as low as your baby will be in his first year of life. You must make the environment safe down there! Cover all of your unused electrical outlets. Small objects and sharp items should be well out of reach. Elevate your houseplants for their safety and the safety of your baby. Some of our most common ones are poisonous.

Beware of long strings, especially with loops, such as drapery pulls or cords attached to blinds. These can hang down and pose great danger.

Preparing the Siblings

You mean this is coming home to stay? Let's get big brother or big sister ready to handle some company!

Is this your first pregnancy? If not, then you may have a big sister and/or a big brother in waiting. They need to be prepared for the change, just like you and your partner. Their world will alter in many ways, and there are certainly things that you can do to help them make the adjustment when the time comes.

First, talk actively about the new baby to come, referring to it as "our baby." This will help to give them a sense of ownership. As your belly grows, you can point to it as the location of the new baby. Depending on their age, siblings may have some input in the choice of names, but be careful as these names may stick!

Check within your community to see if there are any sibling preparation classes. Local hospitals may offer sibling tours. Taking them to your obstetrical appointments will also help them feel more a part of the process—and they will likely get excited to see the baby's heartbeat on the monitor or they will enjoy seeing a sonogram picture.

Remember to have a gift ready, however small, to give to big brother or big sister at the time of the homecoming. This is almost like a peace offering! All of these things will help to lessen sibling rivalry.

Reading books together at home on the subject of expanding the family is very important. These books can be found in the children's section at your local bookstore. As you know, reading together is quality time with any child, and it is especially helpful to read with a child who is about to receive a new sibling.

We Are Having a Baby

As you begin to show, make it clear to the sibling that his baby is in your belly. It will be his baby too. Allow him to touch actively, but gently, and encourage him to talk to the baby-to-be. Keeping your baby's sibling an active part of the pregnancy will pay great dividends once the newborn is at home. Acceptance will come more easily.

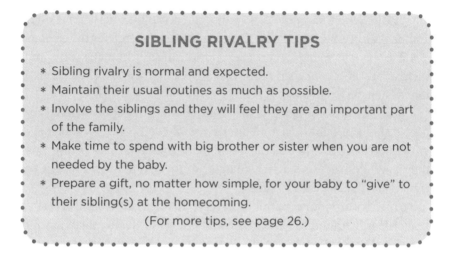

SIBLING RIVALRY TIPS

* Sibling rivalry is normal and expected.
* Maintain their usual routines as much as possible.
* Involve the siblings and they will feel they are an important part of the family.
* Make time to spend with big brother or sister when you are not needed by the baby.
* Prepare a gift, no matter how simple, for your baby to "give" to their sibling(s) at the homecoming.

(For more tips, see page 26.)

Role-playing is a terrific way to help prevent sibling rivalry later. It engenders the care and comfort that we wish to see from the sibling to the new baby. Caring for dolls will model the care and devotion required for the new baby. Teach her to support her doll's head and neck, and to be gentle with her touch.

Practice feedings, burping, changing diapers, and even saying "no" to untoward behavior—not that we need discipline in the first year, but this will resonate with the big brother or sister who receives limits and boundaries from you.

While They Wait

When you are at the hospital, it's best to have loved ones, trusted friends, or babysitters spend time with the sibling(s). Depending on their age, they will be anxiously awaiting your arrival back home, as well as the arrival of their new baby. Those who are caring for them in your absence should be compassionate, reassuring them that everyone is well, and positive regarding all that is happening.

Encourage the caretakers to bring big brother or big sister to the hospital daily to see you and their new baby!

Preparing the Pet

Do you have a beloved pet at home? Your pet is like a sibling, and it needs preparation as well. It is your child too, and deserves some special consideration just as the human siblings do. As you have loved and cared for your pet, or pets, so you will care for your newborn baby. Having a pet is wonderful preparation for having your own children. There are similar changes that a couple goes through when they first get a pet, and raising a child has many common denominators with raising a dog or a cat. For example, we provide proper nutrition, we learn feeding techniques, and we ensure their safety within our homes. Some of us even dress them! We comfort our pets, and we console them when they have been hurt in any way.

Responsible pet owners also find a good veterinarian and take their pets to the doctor's office for routine health care maintenance visits, to be examined and vaccinated, and to receive advice on pet rearing. We take our pets to the doctor when they are ill as well. Even toilet training and discipline are quite similar.

Pet Sibling Rivalry

There are some ways to lessen the sibling rivalry that can exist with pets. First, remember that it is normal and expected, just as it is with human siblings. The family is expanding, and this is quite evident to your dog or cat. As you spend time with them, most pets will sense that something is happening within their "mom." Animals are very intuitive indeed. You must involve them in the process, just as you would a human sibling. Talk about the baby who is soon to come into their lives, especially once you have decided on the baby's name.

They will notice changes in your home; talk about them to your pet as they occur. It is their home too!

Breed familiarity early. It's important to get your pets familiar with their "new sibling" as early as possible. Have dad bring home something from the hospital with the baby's scent on it. Let them smell it. Items that can be brought home from the hospital for this purpose include tee shirts, skull caps, and receiving blankets, all of which have been in contact with your baby's skin. Their sense of smell is powerful, and pets will deposit this, only to recall it once the newborn comes home. Familiarity is important prior to baby's arrival home, for it promotes acceptance in advance. Now you are ready to be one big happy family!

Loving relationships will not fade or leave after the baby comes home, so don't worry. Pets and their families can actually become even closer.

Depending on the pet, reactions can vary. Dogs can become overprotective and maternal, whereas cats may be temporarily aloof or even go into hiding for a period of time.

Preparing the Relatives

This is such a thrilling time in your life, and it is also an incredibly exciting time in the lives of all of your expectant relatives. Whether they will be grandmothers or grandfathers, aunts or uncles, or even close friends, all will be beyond themselves with anticipation for your newborn baby. Even if this is not their first experience with an addition to their family, they will be filled with joy, both for you and for your child.

Family members are almost as anxious and excited as you are. Encourage them to share in the excitement, but without causing you any added stress.

They need to realize that you and your partner need time and space to prepare yourselves, so manage expectations and let everyone know if you want to spend your first few days home from the hospital without any visitors. They can be very helpful in spending time with siblings prior to your delivery day or during your labor. Remember to encourage all of the relatives to be mindful of the sibling or siblings if you have them. Shared attention will ease sibling rivalry, and it will be a good model of sharing for the new brother or sister to see. Children notice everything around them; nothing is lost on them!

There are many benefits for you to enjoy during this process. Your relatives are there for you in all sorts of ways to support you. They will likely shower you with offers to help with childcare at home. And then there is the clothing—they just love to buy clothes for babies!

Require Good Hygiene

Encourage everyone to observe and adopt good hygiene practices, especially before handling and holding the baby. Hand-washing is imperative! If some visitors are in the least bit ill, then they should keep their distance from the newborn until their illness has resolved, as many infections are transmitted via airborne droplets. Most relatives are conscientious about this, but you may have to do some polite policing. Your baby's health depends on this!

Let your relatives revel in the joy of your bringing a beautiful new life into their world . . . they will be lining up to babysit for you!

Accept Their Help

When relatives wish to assist, allow them to be helpful to you, your partner, and your family. Accept graciously. Whether it is an offer to provide a meal, do your laundry, or babysit, it will be helpful to you to lessen your workload in general. Remember that your family members love you . . . just be certain that they know their role is to please you before they please themselves.

CHAPTER ONE

Choosing Your Pediatrician

Choosing a pediatrician will be one of the most important decisions you make regarding your baby's health. This chapter will help you determine who is right for you and what you should ask at prenatal visits with prospective pediatricians. In addition to your pediatrician, you will want to consider the office environment and staff, as well as the doctor's medical philosophy in general and his or her attitude toward medications, vaccinations, and so on. We've included a form with a list of questions to ask the doctor to help you record the differences between pediatricians you interview.

Referral Sources

How should you go about choosing a pediatrician? Valuable referral sources include your family members, your friends, your obstetrician, and even the Internet. This is truly one of the most significant items on your to-do list during your pregnancy. Your relationship with this doctor is a special one, and it will last for a very long time. The doctor you choose will be with you to monitor the overall health, development, and well-being of your children, from infancy to childhood to adolescence to young adulthood.

Pediatricians consider it a privilege to be a part of the family. They are committed not only to monitoring your child's health over time, but also to supporting parents with education. Physicians that choose this specialty love working with children and parents; they find it challenging, stimulating, and rewarding.

Whom should you choose to join you on the journey once you have delivered your baby?

First, ask your loved ones whom they use for pediatric care if they live in the same area as you. Family members are a great source for referrals, because they want what is best for you. Are they happy with the care? Do their children have a good rapport with the pediatrician? Are the doctors accepting new patients? Is the office reasonably close to you?

Next, ask your friends or co-workers how long their children have been patients at their pediatric office. Have their children experienced any illnesses? If so, how were they handled by the doctor and his or her staff? Are mom, dad, and the children happy with the care?

You should ask for a recommendation from your obstetrician, and even ask whom she uses for her children. Feel free to contact your local community hospital for a list of pediatricians on staff.

Techno-savvy folks can consult their computer and use the Internet to gather information on local pediatricians. But the Internet has such a wealth of information that it can also be a bit overwhelming, so try to use it for specific purposes. Seek out websites that may exist for doctors and their offices that are under your consideration. Gather information about training and any current academic affiliations they may have. They may be involved in teaching their specialty to medical students, interns, and residents at nearby schools of medicine. Use the Internet for information on a physician's credentials, academic affiliations, hospital privileges, and any special interests or specialties that he or she may have. Be careful not to consult sites that rate physicians, as they post anything and everything, both positive and negative. The information is inconsistent; it may be totally false. Such information may seem beneficial during your search, but these sites take no responsibility for their content and do not support any of the information as factual.

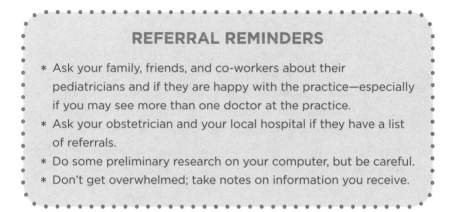

REFERRAL REMINDERS

* Ask your family, friends, and co-workers about their pediatricians and if they are happy with the practice—especially if you may see more than one doctor at the practice.
* Ask your obstetrician and your local hospital if they have a list of referrals.
* Do some preliminary research on your computer, but be careful.
* Don't get overwhelmed; take notes on information you receive.

The Prenatal Visit

After you have received recommendations, it is important to avail yourself | 3
of the opportunity to meet with some of the doctors. Most pediatric offices offer a prenatal visit, which usually consists of a face-to-face meeting with the doctor without fee or obligation. The time is best spent seeking answers to questions, both general and specific. No question is too silly to ask. Don't be shy. Try not to treat this time as a formal interview, lest you invoke a particular physician's defenses. Rather, use this visit to see if you feel comfortable with the doctor.

It's helpful to have your partner with you for the prenatal visits so that you can compare notes and feelings about the meetings afterward. You will sit with the doctors in their offices, and you should get a sense of their responsiveness to your concerns. The right pediatrician is someone who will both hear you and listen to you. You will need his or her support and education as parents.

Some pediatricians may have literature to give you to take home and read. Be careful not to read too much . . . the amount of information available can be overwhelming! Again, make time to meet with doctors so that you will be prepared to choose this important and trusted friend. There are many things to consider as you schedule your prenatal visit. Are you comfortable with the setting and with the doctor's style? First impressions can be meaningful. If he is able to join you for the meeting, is your partner as comfortable as you are? You must consider his feelings as well. Feel free to bring a written list of questions so that you won't forget to ask the things you have been wondering about. Also ask about the doctor's medical philosophy in general.

QUESTIONS TO ASK

* What happens when I get to the hospital?
* When will our baby first be examined?
* What can we expect from our pediatrician during the hospital stay?
* What can we expect from the doctor's office over time?
* How do you feel about the use of medication in general?
* Do you follow the recommended vaccine schedule?

Take a Tour

A visit to the pediatric office will be helpful to both of you as you decide which doctor and office to choose. Are you greeted warmly by the office staff and by the doctor? Do the nurses seem approachable and knowledgeable? Are you offered a tour of the office and the exam rooms? Is the office setting child-friendly? Is it bright, cozy, and comforting?

Ask the Doctor

The visit should be informative and educational, so don't hesitate to ask all of your questions. The pediatrician that cares will address any question you bring, no matter how simple or silly it seems to you. Remember that pediatricians are accustomed to educating parents about wellness, illness, development, and so on. They are trained to be a source of information for you.

Your Pediatrician's Medical Philosophy

How does your doctor feel about medication, and how do you feel about it?

The use of medication today is a hot topic, and a valid one to be discussed with any prospective pediatrician. This is the doctor you will entrust with the ongoing care of your child, and whom you will refer to for his or her advice regarding the use of medication.

Please look for a physician who has an academic philosophy when it comes to advising or administering medications. An academic philosophy is judicious. That is to say that medication should only be utilized when it is truly needed. Rest, fluids (especially chicken soup!), and tender loving care will get most of us through most illnesses. On the other hand, when medication is indicated, it should be used definitively and in the appropriate dosage for the correct duration required. Medication is overused by patients and overprescribed by some physicians, and this is not what you need. You should certainly ask the doctors at your prenatal visits about their feelings with regard to medication use.

Ask the doctor at this visit if she waits a period of time before using new medications on the market. Most pediatricians are well read and trust that the appropriate studies have been carried out prior to the FDA approving a particular medication for widespread use. Doctors follow guidelines that include age indications. They are careful not to do anything that will harm your children.

It is also important to ask about the vaccination policy at the pediatric office. Most pediatricians follow the current recommendations from the American Academy of Pediatrics (AAP). The recommendations emanate from the foremost leaders in pediatric infectious disease, who guide the research in this field of pediatric medicine. They have no hidden agenda; the optimum health and safety of all children is their goal.

Your pediatrician should be willing, able, and available to discuss the currently recommended vaccine protocol and to answer any questions you may have pertaining to this. In particular, there has been much controversy over the past ten years with regard to the risk-to-benefit ratio of certain vaccines, with possible implications for the development of our children. Also, preservatives formerly utilized in many vaccines were found to cause elevated levels of mercury in some individuals, leading to adverse effects on learning. All of these issues, well founded or not, should be discussed with the doctor.

To Vaccinate or Not to Vaccinate?

There is still a good degree of controversy regarding the vaccine protocol.

Most pediatricians follow the AAP recommended guidelines. These can be found at www.aap.org. Though no real evidence exists to warrant any alteration in the schedule, some parents wish to separate vaccines by coming to the office more often; more days with fewer vaccines per day, resulting in the same reception over time.

Office and Staff

When you choose your pediatrician, you also need to consider his office in the decision-making process. Even though finding the right doctor for your baby is paramount, you'll want to achieve a certain comfort level at the pediatric office as well. Medical offices and practices vary greatly.

QUESTIONS TO ASK PROSPECTIVE PEDIATRICIANS

What are the office hours?

What is the average wait time in the office?

Is the office open for weekend hours?

Is the office open for evening hours?

Who shares the on-call hours with my doctor when the office is closed for the day?

How do you feel about the use of medication?

Do you follow the currently recommended vaccine protocol?

Will you vary the vaccine schedule if requested?

Will you refuse to care for patients who refuse to vaccinate their children?

Some are small and independent, and others are in large buildings as part of multispecialty groups.

Regardless of size, it's important to find an office that is clean, up-to-date, and conducive to children playing in the waiting room. Most pediatric offices are decorated in a child-friendly manner. The pediatric staff should be warm and welcoming, patient and comfortable with children of all ages.

Clerical staff meet and greet, take care of all appointment needs, as well as receive insurance information from all patients. Pediatric nurses are devoted to the care of newborns through young adults. They should relate well to all of the patients. The pediatric office and practice is dependent on the expertise of the nursing staff. Nurses give medical advice by phone, as trained by the physicians. This allows the doctors to stay on schedule with patient visits. As in all fields, nurses know their limits, and they won't hesitate to check with the doctors on a given issue.

You may have been told to look for a pediatric office with two separate waiting rooms—one for well visits, and one for ill visits. Don't be overly concerned with this. First, most pediatric offices do not have separate waiting rooms. Second, remember that the air is shared in the halls and examination rooms. Most viral shedding is airborne, so exposure is not eliminated. Finally, patients who are present for their well-child visit may be ill at the same time.

Pediatric Phone Advice

Pediatric nurses give phone advice during the workday. They know their limits and check with the doctor as needed. No question is too small, so don't hesitate to call. The nurse can be very helpful in deciding whether an office visit is necessary.

Kid-Friendly—Parent-Friendly

Pediatric staff members usually function as an extended family. They should make you and your child feel right at home. Clerical staff handle appointments, insurance needs, prior authorizations, and patient medical records. The office may have electronic medical records (EMR), utilizing today's technology for improved patient care. Look for a feeling of comfort, beginning with your entrance into an office and ending with your exit.

Large and Small Offices

Office sizes and practices may vary, but pediatric care should not. In any setting, pediatricians are devoted to their patients, whether they be infants, children, adolescents, or young adults. The key is to find the office and the pediatrician with whom you are most comfortable. The relationship could potentially last for twenty-one years. In some pediatric practices, physicians share the families, but most have their own primary patient population. When this is the practice style, one pediatrician is the primary provider of care for the children of a family, but the children are usually exposed to the other doctors in the practice when their primary pediatrician is unavailable. This is valuable because both parents and children will be comfortable seeing their doctor's colleagues.

Is it Nearby?

Is the pediatric office in your neighborhood? If not, is it easy to find? It need not be in your immediate vicinity, although most parents don't wish to be too far away from their doctor's office or their local community hospital. Some pediatric offices are connected to large tertiary care centers or attached to medical schools, especially in urban settings. This is just another variation in the theme that you may be introduced to as you visit offices.

On-Call Coverage

Physicians are available around the clock to care for and advise their patients. This comes with the territory, and here is how it works: Most offices have routine daytime office hours. When the office has closed for the day, the phones are turned over to an answering service. After-hours phone calls are delivered to the doctor who is "on call" that evening. When a doctor is on call, he is available through the night until the next morning when the office has reopened.

Pediatricians, like other physicians, generally share these nights with several colleagues during the week and the weekend. This allows them to be on call intermittently, but not every night. If they did not share the after-hours duty, they would surely be too fatigued to take good care of your children. Therefore, your own pediatrician may not be the doctor who responds to your evening call, but an equally trained pediatrician will be available to you, and it will be a colleague who is trusted to give you appropriate advice.

When you make an after-hours call, the physician on the phone will take a history and ask questions that will allow her to make her best judgment call, given that she has to advise you over the phone and not in person. Advice may include supportive care at home or encouragement to go to the nearest emergency department for evaluation. The advice depends on the history, or story, if you will, that is received. When you are speaking to the on-call pediatrician, be certain to let her know your child's medical background, especially if you are not speaking to your primary provider. This will allow the doctor to best guide you. Such particulars include the baby's age, weight, and any pertinent medical history that exists (for example, frequent ear infections, asthma, allergies, and so on).

Although after-hours calls are meant to be for urgent issues, or for guidance regarding acute illnesses, when you are a new parent it may not be that clear to you. Err on the side of caution. Pediatricians are patient and committed to education, and they are accustomed to this. With time and experience, parents become more discerning as to what necessitates a call.

CHAPTER TWO

What to Expect in the Hospital

What happens when the baby comes? Your relationship with your pediatrician is about to begin! When you have been admitted to the labor and delivery suite, one of the first questions you will be asked is the name of your pediatrician. Once you have delivered your baby, your pediatrician will be notified. Of course, the neonatal nursing staff will have attended to and assessed the baby initially, but the first full physical examination by the pediatrician will take place within twelve to twenty-four hours, depending on your time of delivery. If you deliver the baby by day, your pediatrician may come to examine the baby after office hours that evening. If you deliver overnight, he or she will arrive first thing in the morning.

After completing the examination, he or she will visit your room and tell you all about the baby. This is an exciting time, and you may be exhausted, but pay attention to each detail of the assessment as it is described for you. It's best when your partner is with you, as you may be tired or still under the effects of medication, particularly if you have required a cesarean section for delivery. Your pediatrician will describe the examination, including any findings that are of concern. Thankfully, this is uncommon. You will have a beautiful new baby girl or boy!

At the time of delivery, the nursing staff will dry and stimulate your baby and suction the nose and mouth to relieve him of amniotic fluid and saliva. They will assign him Apgar scores at one minute and five minutes of life. This is a judge of the baby's initial status, and it considers heart rate, muscle tone, reflex irritability, color, and breathing. Each quality is scored up to two points, and rarely does the amount total ten. Apgar scores of seven to nine are quite acceptable and denote very good first function for your baby.

Checking In at the Hospital

When you are in labor, you will be checking in at the labor and delivery section of the hospital. Of course, if you have a scheduled c-section, you will arrive at the appropriately scheduled time. Remember to have your medical information and insurance information handy so that the process will be smooth and efficient. You will be asked the name of your pediatrician of choice. The labor and delivery nursing staff will make you feel comfortable as you settle in.

Most deliveries are without complication. Your hospital, doctors, and staff are prepared for any departure from the routine.

If you or your baby has a special need, seen or unforeseen, the staff will be ready to care for you both as needed. If the baby has any difficulty during delivery, it will be attended to immediately; this may include temporary monitoring or even admission and care in the neonatal intensive care unit (NICU).

Babies that will require the NICU include those that are premature and those that have any respiratory distress following their delivery.

Meet Your New Doctor

Your baby is here and it's time for her to meet your pediatrician. This is when the first full physical examination takes place, usually in the newborn nursery. After the examination, your pediatrician will speak to you about the baby. You may still be in your delivery room, the recovery room (following a c-section), or already settled in your postpartum room. The doctor will reassure you and fill you in on his findings, including the baby's length, head circumference, and any significant findings on physical examination.

Each morning that you are in the hospital, your pediatrician will be "making rounds." He will examine your baby and then come to talk with you. At this time, you will be given a report regarding the baby's exam, daily weight, how well she eliminated (urine and stool), and any other issues. The doctor will then share some information regarding the nuances of newborns and their care. This is a time for education and an opportunity for you to ask any questions you may have.

Newborn Behaviors

The pediatrician has obligations to you in the hospital, and these include examining your baby daily, reporting all of the baby's daily statistics to you, and sharing information with you. There is time to do this, although hospital stays vary. We are bound to insurance company coverage, which is generally two allowable days following a vaginal delivery, and four days following a cesarean section. During these days in the hospital, the time that your pediatrician spends with you is invaluable. She will share any necessary medical information that pertains to your baby, and you will learn about the most common newborn behaviors.

Every newborn baby is special and unique, but they all exhibit behaviors that need no treatment. Your pediatrician will explain the benign and expected nature of these behaviors. Armed with this knowledge, you and your partner will feel reassured, and you can then relieve all of the baby's fans, who may be worried as well. You may wish to take notes about the things you learn, both to remember subsequently and to refer to when sharing with your family, friends, and loved ones.

One of the most common newborn behaviors is called periodic breathing of the newborn. This is more common in the premature infant but is also normal in the full-term infant. Unbeknownst to you, the baby slows or stops his breathing pattern for a short period of time—seconds. When the baby begins the breathing pattern again, he or she gathers several breaths and then sighs. There is no distress or color change, just the brief change in pattern. Then the baby is quiet again. No worries.

Communication

How do newborns communicate with us? They tend to express themselves vocally and with their body language. You will become more familiar with your baby and his communication with you as each day goes by. You will come to know him better than anyone else as you connect daily. Crying is their main form of communication, but it doesn't mean that they are sad or in pain. It's the way they talk to us. It may mean that they are hungry, need to be changed, or simply need to be held.

Babies also communicate via body language all the time. When babies are unhappy they will be unsettled or even noticeably uncomfortable. When babies are content, they are quiet. The Moro reflex, or "startle reflex," is normal and neurologic; it comes from the brain. Your baby's arms will fly up with hands and fingers outstretched, as if she is frightened, and her lips may quiver. All is settled within seconds. This is not a seizure; it is quite normal.

Sneezing and Hiccups

Sneezing and hiccups are both common during the first two months of life, and they are both normal behaviors. With a sneeze, your baby is clearing secretions. She is not cold, and she does not as yet have a cold. Hiccups occur in utero and then once baby is born. No need to stop a feeding; you may feed through these and they will stop after about thirty minutes. No treatment is needed for sneezing or hiccups. They are normal behaviors.

Eye Deviation

Oh no! My baby has crooked eyes! What happened? Not to worry—this is normal too. Newborns are born with weak extra-ocular eye musculature.

This means that they can deviate any which way but loose! They can look cross-eyed for up to six months. Once the muscles tighten with time, they track together as you would expect. Only rarely does a deviation persist, leading to a consultation with a pediatric ophthalmologist. Let your newborn stare at his nose for now . . . it is normal.

Eye Color and Vision

Pediatricians are often asked about the baby's eye color. Most babies are born with slate blue eyes, but this doesn't usually last. Brown is genetically dominant, and blue is recessive. Whatever color they are going to have, it may take an entire year to see the exact hue that they will be keeping, so please be patient.

As far as visual acuity is concerned, experts reassure us that newborns can indeed see, but that vision is not yet 20/20. In fact, it may be 20/800! They can see and focus perhaps eight inches away, and beyond that they are said to be able to see shadows. Of course, their vision improves over time.

Newborns are accustomed to darkness in utero. Therefore, they initially keep their eyes closed, especially in bright light. This is normal. As they adjust over time, you will see their eyes open more often. They can see you up close and personal, perhaps focusing at seven or eight inches away. Visual acuity increases with each month; they will see you across the room by four months of age.

If you notice that one eye (or both) is a bit runny with clear tears, it is possible that she has been born with a blocked tear duct. This is not uncommon, and it is called dacryostenosis. You did not cause this; it is idiopathic, meaning there is no known cause. It happens more often in one eye only, and it usually resolves within the first year of life. Your pediatrician may advise massage over the tear duct if this persists.

15

Umbilical Cord Care

Cord care is easy. The umbilical cord is moist and off-white at birth. Wharton's jelly protects the umbilical vessels within the cord. The cord will be clamped directly following birth; this keeps the cord from bleeding out. The clamp will be removed before you go home. The cord may be blue from a drying agent or dye used in some nurseries.

Simply use a Q-tip and rubbing alcohol around the base of the cord where it meets the skin three to four times daily. This will dry the system and keep it clean, and it should fall off between ten and twenty days. Then you can do immersion baths instead of sponge bathing. An added benefit to using the alcohol is that it will stimulate your baby to awaken for her daytime feedings so try this at feeding time. It doesn't hurt but it's cold as it dries. What a wake-up call!

TIPS FOR THE TIPS

* It's best to do cord and circumcision care during the day, as we don't want to perform stimulating procedures on the baby overnight. We want the baby to sleep!
* Don't pull on the cord; it won't come off, but it will be uncomfortable for the baby.
* Use Vaseline, Aquaphor ointment, or antibiotic ointment for the tip of the penis. Infection is rare, so you do not necessarily have to use an antibiotic ointment. Three times daily will do.
* The cord will fall off—the penis will not!

Circumcision Care

If you have decided to circumcise your baby boy, the care is quite simple and easy.

Use an ointment to lubricate the tip (called the glans penis) three to four times a day for just one week. The purpose is to prevent the moist healing tip from sticking to the diaper. As it heals, it is common for the tip to look a bit soupy, with yellow patches. This is granulation tissue, the normal healing process, and it is not a sign of infection.

All About the Skin

The skin of the newborn baby is indeed soft and smooth, and it is lovely to touch. Your baby needs to have your touch, and he will come to know his mother's touch like no other. This daily frequent contact will bring comfort that will last throughout his life.

Your baby has been immersed for months in amniotic fluid, so her skin will appear quite dry to you. This is completely normal, so don't worry. Because her skin has been swimming in fluid for so long, it must dry out. That's why it is dry and peels in the first days of life. One can even see cracks and bleeding in some areas, such as around the ankles, especially with ankle bands for identification and security.

Feel free to moisturize your baby's skin, but be aware that it is not medically necessary. We are bothered by their dryness, but they are not. If you do moisturize their skin, be certain to use safe, hypoallergenic, and fragrance-free products. Your baby already smells good enough!

IT'S A MYTH!

Fearful relatives may make comments or pressure you to cover your baby's ears or to be careful not to allow any water to enter the ear canal. Break the myth: You do not have to worry about this at all. Water is necessary for bathing, and you will want to bathe and cleanse your baby's scalp and hair. Water enters the ear canal, travels up to the eardrum, and then turns around to travel back out. Water in (and out) of the ear canal can actually assist the travel of wax on its way out of the ear canal. Water will not cause ear infections in your baby. The middle ear infection occurs on the other side of the eardrum.

Birthmarks, Strange Color, and Skin Rashes

Congenital birthmarks occur, and these are usually benign or harmless. Most of these birthmarks are temporary, and you will watch them fade away over time. A congenital birthmark can be flat and brown in color and is called a pigmented nevus. Others are red in color, such as a port wine stain. These two types of birthmarks are uncommon, and they remain. Your pediatrician and a dermatologist will monitor them.

A flame nevus is a benign pink or salmon-colored patch that many babies are born with. The most commonly affected areas of the skin are the eyelids, the bridge of the nose, the forehead, and the nape of the neck. The lay terms for these are "angel kisses" when they appear on the face, and "stork bites" when they appear on the neck. These birthmarks require no treatment. Those on the face fade and leave within two years, and those on the neck may remain forever.

Acrocyanosis is a normal finding in almost every newborn baby. It looks worrisome because we expect our babies to be pink all over. This is a blue or purple discoloration on the palms of the hands and the soles of the feet. The palms and soles may also feel a bit cooler than the rest of your baby's skin. This is also normal, and it will not last more than a few days. No treatment is needed for acrocyanosis. Tell your concerned family members that it is temporary!

Erythema toxicum (or E-tox) is a very benign newborn rash that appears as single pink blotches with a small, raised lighter dot in the middle. Actually, these blotches resemble flea bites! They can appear anywhere on the body, and they may come and go for several weeks. They go unnoticed by your baby, are asymptomatic, and require no treatment at all.

Milia are small white dots or cysts, usually seen on the nose and occasionally on the face. They are hormonally induced. Most babies have these, and they go away within months. Neonatal or infant acne appears on the face of some infants at one to two weeks of life, not right away. Also hormonally induced, these lesions look just like teenage acne, but require no treatment and leave within weeks on their own.

Skin Irritations

Newborn baby skin is new to the environment and no longer protected by your womb. Their skin is tender and is susceptible to becoming irritated. Irritation can occur whenever skin is exposed to surfaces, particularly rough ones, such as a father's whiskers. Skin can also become irritated simply through contact with the nursing mother's breast. This is expected. Cheeks and chins are the most commonly irritated areas of the skin, because the baby must make contact as she feeds. Unless the irritation is severe, your baby will not experience pain from it. Feel free to use a hypoallergenic cream, lotion, or ointment on the irritated skin. Moisturizing will soothe the irritated skin, and it will soothe your feelings and the worries of relatives! Of course, every infant is unique in this regard. Some babies don't get irritated at all.

19

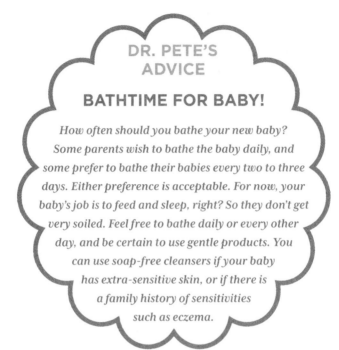

DR. PETE'S ADVICE

BATHTIME FOR BABY!

How often should you bathe your new baby?
Some parents wish to bathe the baby daily, and
some prefer to bathe their babies every two to three
days. Either preference is acceptable. For now, your
baby's job is to feed and sleep, right? So they don't get
very soiled. Feel free to bathe daily or every other
day, and be certain to use gentle products. You
can use soap-free cleansers if your baby
has extra-sensitive skin, or if there is
a family history of sensitivities
such as eczema.

If there is a family history of sensitive skin, your baby may have an increased risk of being sensitive as well. Only time will tell. Please let your pediatrician know of any history of eczema or psoriasis, especially in you or the baby's father, so that you can be on the alert for this together.

Also, babies can easily scratch themselves with their fingernails. This is superficial, so there is no need for you to panic! Again, they are not bothered, and no treatment is indicated. All of these irritations bother parents more than they bother babies, so don't fret. However, we can be preventive with attentive skin and nail care. Skin infections from any of these irritations are rare. Fingernails grow rapidly, whereas toenails grow slowly. You will find that the fingers need attention twice as often as the toes. You may file nails downward with an emery board or use a curved scissor with a blunt end. Refrain from using infant-size clippers, as these can pinch the skin.

Your baby may have prominent veins on his scalp or face. This is a normal finding, particularly in babies whose coloration is lighter or fairer than most. As babies grow, so does the thickness of their skin—they will grow into those veins!

Yellow Belly Blues

Jaundice is common and peaks during the third day of life, decreasing over the next several weeks. Jaundice is a yellow discoloration of the skin that most babies display. It begins in the sclera (white part of the eyes), and if it progresses, it includes the face, proceeding downward toward the chest. Newborns have too many red blood cells, so they break and release the substance bilirubin. This gets processed in the liver. Bilirubin goes from the liver to the gastrointestinal tract and out with the stool. Most babies can't keep up with the process, so the traffic jam causes the bilirubin to increase in the bloodstream, and it manifests as a yellow pigmentation on their skin. Babies that feed well have less jaundice.

Hyperbilirubinemia, or increased jaundice, occurs in the premature infant, during infection, dehydration, and when baby's blood type disagrees with yours.

Your pediatrician will monitor this closely for you in the hospital and also in his office.

Sucking Blisters

Look closely at your baby's sweet lips, and you will see that they appear wrinkled. This is a sucking blister. Most blisters are uncomfortable to us, but sucking blisters are not painful for your baby. These blisters are circumferential (all around the lips), and they are the direct result of all of that sucking. No prevention, no pain, no treatment, and no cure, other than tincture of time!

Getting Ready to Leave the Hospital

As you prepare to be discharged from the hospital, you will be considering how to dress your beautiful baby. You will undoubtedly receive lots of advice from well-intentioned relatives, and perhaps from hospital staff members. Remember that it is really simple, and not an issue that should make you anxious. Infants—even newborns—adjust to their environment, just as we do. It is important to keep them warm and dry directly following birth as they are first exposed to extra-uterine life.

The neonatal nursing staff will take care of this for your baby. It is wise to keep their beanie caps on their heads for the first twenty hours of life to prevent heat loss, as the surface area of skin on the head is actually quite large. Hats are helpful in the winter, especially if the baby's hair is sparse. Otherwise, they can feel uncomfortable with extremes, just as we can. So be practical. Keep your baby warm but not overheated. Watch out for heat rash. If this occurs, it means you used too many layers, causing the baby to sweat, which causes heat rash.

Use the "one layer more" philosophy as your guide to dressing your baby. Dress him with one layer more than you would use to dress yourself, and he will be both safe and comfortable. This applies to any season of the year.

HOT OR COLD?

Your hospital room in the postpartum ward will have a thermostat so that your room will be comfortable for you. The temperature in the hospital nursery will also be well controlled for your baby's comfort. At your home, be certain not to change the climate that you enjoyed prior to having your baby. You came first. Maintain your usual home temperature, and dress your baby appropriately. It is really that simple. Enjoy your home and your family!

Swaddling

Newborn babies are swaddled in the hospital nursery. This keeps them snug and warm and comfortable. Swaddling in the first days of life allows them to feel secure, as if they are still in your womb. Swaddling thereafter is not necessary, unless your baby seems to prefer it. Some infants love this tight feeling. However, some babies hate to be swaddled. This simply means your baby does not like restriction. Both tendencies are normal; you will come to know what your baby prefers as you get to know each other with each passing day. If you swaddle your baby, simply be mindful to count all of the layers so that she is not overheated.

Have Car Seat, Will Travel!

Going out in public with your new baby is indeed a reality! Despite much controversy, it is healthy to be out in the fresh air, as long as the baby is dressed appropriately. You need not be sequestered in your home for days, weeks, or months. The only restriction is large public places, such as malls, busy restaurants, or grocery stores. Your baby should not be exposed to these settings for two months.

You are now going to leave the hospital, and you must protect your baby from all harm. This begins with the car seat. Do your research ahead of time regarding the different types of car seat systems available on the market. Prepare ahead like the Boy Scouts do! You will find infant-only seats as well as convertible models. Infant-only seats are smaller, and they usually click into a base that may be left securely in the car. Convertible seats are larger and don't have carrying handles, but they can be used later, forward facing, when your child is older. The convertible car seat is useful for larger babies because of its increased rear-facing weight. Some car seats require you to utilize the car seat belt for secure restraint.

Cars manufactured after 2002 may have the LATCH system. This stands for Lower Anchors and Tethers for Children, and it is a secure attachment system that alleviates the need to use the seat belt on the car safety seat. Your car seat and your car must both have this system. If they do, the car safety seat will directly attach to the LATCH receptacles, or anchors, which are found in the backseat of the car. Rear facing is mandatory and is now recommended until your baby is two years old. This is the safest position for infants. Many parents wish to sit in the backseat with their new baby to watch her and to be certain that she is safe. Feel free to sit with your baby, but know that it is not necessary as long as she is comfortable and secure in her car safety seat. Rest assured that she will enjoy a safe ride home with her parents, even if you are in the front seat.

Your baby's safety is vital; read, practice, and prepare. Before bringing your baby to the car for the first time, be certain to double- or triple-check the car safety system. Harness straps need to be secured at or below your baby's shoulders. The usual five-point restraint includes a strap that rises between your baby's legs and attaches to a central latch, connecting the waist and shoulder straps. Read the manual carefully so that you don't miss anything. Keep the manual in the car glove box. Be certain your baby is comfortable, safe, and secure. Settle the baby's head and neck comfortably and securely using the molded fabric that came with your car seat. Always drive safely. You are carrying the most precious cargo.

CAR SEAT SAFETY TIPS

* Parents should know how to use the car safety seat system.
* Hand-me-downs are great, but be careful with car seats. They must be up-to-date and in perfect shape.
* Rear facing is the safest position and is a must for your new baby; it is now recommended through age two.
* Be sure not to place the car seat in an elevated spot (a counter, for example) with your baby in it. It's best to leave it on the floor, avoiding accidental falls and injury.

CHAPTER THREE

Home, James!

It's time to come home to the big brother or big sister, as well as your pet.

Little things mean a lot right now. Every small consideration will make a big difference. You should enter and greet the sibling without the baby. Let someone follow you in with the new baby. Have a gift ready to give to big brother or sister from the new baby. A gift exchange goes a long way. This is such an exciting time in your life, and it is equally exciting to your new baby's siblings. Depending on the brother or sister and his or her age, you may not encounter an easy and instant acceptance. Hopefully you have prepared siblings for the change as much as possible by reading with them and actively speaking with them about the new baby to come. They may have helped you with input on the name, or on the colors of the nursery. You probably have had big brother or sister talking to the baby through your belly. All of these considerations will help them adjust.

Sibling Rivalry

Sibling rivalry can begin before the baby is born, but it usually begins once the new baby has arrived home. Once the baby enters your lives, you may begin to notice signs of jealousy. After all, thus far your older child has been the focus of your lives. He may be very upset with you, not the baby. Some will act out in ways you have not anticipated—some may be aggressive, and others may show signs of regression in their behavior. Again, this is expected, but the response that you give to the new sibling is important, as we don't wish for the behavior to continue for long. It's best to accept it as normal and to allow your child to be honest about his feelings, but be careful not to give the behavior much attention.

Remember basic psychology here. You should give your child praise and positive attention for the behavior that you want to continue, such as helpfulness, politeness, gentle touch with the new baby, and so on. The older sibling will see that she receives attention for these behaviors and will be more apt to reproduce them. You should set aside some time to spend alone with the big brother or big sister. Quality time with mom and dad, with the new baby and without the new baby, is vital.

Siblings need to take part in the care of their new baby, and they usually want to help. They will feel needed and wanted if they are included. Give them simple tasks, such as retrieving a blanket or choosing baby's outfit. It's not always easy to involve a sibling. It can actually add to your work, but it will surely ease the rivalry for the sibling.

Sibling rivalry can be frustrating, but a commonsense approach will lessen the trauma for everyone. With time, even the most jealous of siblings will adjust to the new family order with the bonds of love.

ADDITIONAL SIBLING RIVALRY TIPS

* Always listen and acknowledge the sibling's feelings.
* Maintain the same rules as always. Otherwise, she may learn to manipulate.
* Include the sibling in your daily routine as your helper.
* Set aside some one-on-one time every day.
* Encourage the relatives to pay enough attention to the sibling.
* Make sure that the new big brother or big sister is always supervised and gentle with the new baby.

(See also page xvi in the Introduction.)

Create a Night Sleeper

Sleep is essential for everyone, especially your new baby. Newborns need at least sixteen hours of sleep per day—often much more. Initially, it seems that all they do is feed and sleep. The newborn infant stomach is small, and frequent feedings are necessary. This leads to regular awakening out of hunger, with short intervals between feedings, which spells exhaustion for you!

Your baby will probably be sleepier during the day and more awake at night in the first weeks of life. This is because you were "rocking" him by day during your pregnancy. When they are born, babies are accustomed to this activity and are therefore quieter in the daytime. It's often difficult to arouse them for feedings by day. At night they are more often awake since you were quiet in the evening and through the night during pregnancy. All of this will change with time, but you must be patient and follow some simple guidelines.

We must undo this pattern in order to have a night sleeper. It can be accomplished lovingly and without harm. First, be prepared for feedings on demand, which could mean every two to three hours initially. Treat daytime as it is, with a normal amount of activity, noise, light, and routine. Feed your baby every three hours during the day, unless she demands it sooner. Treat nighttime as it should be for your baby—dark, quiet, and boring. With time, the baby will get used to a bright, active day and a dark, boring night. Feed only on demand at night.

Establish a bedtime routine from the start. His sleep intervals will increase, aided by a larger stomach capacity with a greater volume of food as he grows. Most babies will be sleeping through the night between three and five months of age.

Day Is Day

Treat daytime as you always would. Keep your baby with you, not in a quiet place. Arouse her to feed if it has been three hours since the last feeding.

This is not always easy. On-demand feeding is the rule, but don't exceed those three hours in between. Routine noise, light, siblings, family, and friends are all fine during the daytime. Over time, your baby will adjust to become more wakeful during the day.

It's important for you to rest when the baby is sleeping. You need to be well for your baby. Fight the urge to spring into action and "get things done" while he sleeps. The laundry can wait! You must rest! When it seems difficult to arouse your baby for a daytime feeding, unswaddle him and tickle his feet, and stroke the mandible (jaw) to help awaken him. Remember that routine is good. You can have on-demand feeding and still foster a routine that will be accepted.

Night Is Night

Never wake a baby after eight o'clock in the evening. Nighttime is the right time to forget that three-hour daytime sleep limitation. After the clock strikes eight, only feed your baby when she awakens to demand it, which can be quite often in the first week or two of life. Again, routine is good even now. An evening bath, lotion, song, or prayer is a good thing by eight at night.

At night, keep a night-light on for your safety, but no popcorn and movies. Be boring overnight and she will be sleeping through soon!

Back to Sleep

Since 1992, the American Academy of Pediatrics has advised that infants should sleep supine, or on their back, for naps and bedtime. The campaign for infants to sleep on their back has resulted in a great reduction in deaths from SIDS (Sudden Infant Death Syndrome). Also try to alternate the position of your baby's head so as to help prevent positional molding called plagiocephaly.

Keep the bassinet or crib free of blankets, toys, and pillows for now Ask all of your baby's caretakers to do as you do.

Why Do They Cry?

Crying doesn't always mean we are hurting or sad, and so it is with your new baby. It is indeed one of the ways that newborns speak to us. Early on, it simply means that it is time for his feeding. As you get to know him, you will become accustomed to his needs and wants. Often, you may even be able to identify the issue by the quality of the cry. There may be a distinct cry for hunger and a different cry for the need to be changed or held. Check for an eyelash in the eye, or a hair wrapped around a finger or toe. These uncommon occurrences can make a baby cry. When a baby is in pain, his cry is often high-pitched, loud, and unrelenting. You will come to know the difference with time. If it's feeding time, you know what to do. If he needs a diaper change, he will be content following the drill. Sometimes they need a feeding and also a diaper change!

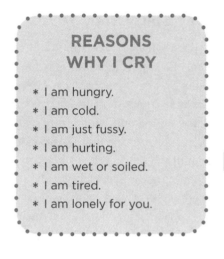

REASONS WHY I CRY

* I am hungry.
* I am cold.
* I am just fussy.
* I am hurting.
* I am wet or soiled.
* I am tired.
* I am lonely for you.

29

Babies can cry when they are overtired or overhandled by many relatives in a short period of time. Investigate whether a sibling has bothered her lovingly, such as with an inquisitive finger to the baby's eye! If your baby begins to cry frequently at around two weeks of life, and also draws up her legs as if in discomfort, with or without extra gas, she may have colic. Colic causes abdominal discomfort of varying degrees, more often in the evening, and is a common cause of crying in babies. The baby who cries for hours and seems inconsolable is of great concern. Thankfully, serious infection is uncommon in infants, but it does occur. If your baby cries more than two or three hours total in a day, a medical issue may be the culprit. If a baby is hot or cold to touch, take her temperature. This is important in early infancy.

If your baby is inconsolable, bring her to your pediatrician for evaluation. He will do a thorough examination and seek a cause for your baby's distress. Then he will advise you of the need for any intervention.

The Spitty Baby

Spitty babies may be simply spitty, or they may have an allergy or reflux, but the vomiting infant may be sick. A baby that is vomiting is of great concern. A cause must be determined by your pediatrician before the baby becomes dehydrated. This can occur quickly in the young infant. After ruling out a milk protein allergy or a bacterial infection, one must consider pyloric stenosis, especially if your baby has episodes of projectile vomiting. Beyond the wet burp, this is forceful vomiting that can send a feeding several feet away. This is disconcerting to see, but don't panic. Of course, bring your baby to the pediatrician for evaluation.

Pyloric stenosis is a narrowing of the pylorus, which is the opening between the stomach and the small intestine. A stenotic or narrowed pylorus is due to a thickening of its muscle. This is rare and has no known cause. It occurs more often in boys, and the symptoms usually appear at three to four weeks of age. The hallmark symptom is projectile vomiting; a feeding will build up without easy flow through the pylorus, eventually coming back out of the mouth. This is a mechanical phenomenon and does not typically give a baby pain. The feedings simply come back up shortly after being received. It may not occur after every feeding, and you may see a wavelike motion of the abdomen just before the vomiting episode.

Unlike babies with infections, those with pyloric stenosis are hungry right away after vomiting and want to feed again. They don't generally appear ill. Your pediatrician should immediately evaluate your baby if he is projectile vomiting, and she may order an abdominal ultrasound to make the diagnosis. The treatment is a pyloromyotomy, or opening of the muscle, which is done surgically by a pediatric surgeon.

To Burp or Not to Burp

Burping is important for relieving the air that comes with swallowing. Burp vigorously; your baby will enjoy the vibration as she did in utero when you were walking. Some of a feeding may come up with a burp. It's a small amount, and it is called a wet burp. If a baby is consistently spitty within an hour of a feeding, this may be an indication of more than just a wet burp.

Is it an Allergy?

Some babies spit because they are reacting to the feeding they receive. They may feed well, but then reject some or all of the feeding. If you are breast-feeding, enjoy all foods, but in moderation. If you have food sensitivities, of course avoid such foods in your own diet. Food allergy is uncommon in infancy, but it does occur. It is often familial. Ask your relatives about their history. Your baby may simply be adjusting to first feedings, but there's a chance he may have a milk protein allergy. Ask your pediatrician about this.

31

IT'S A MYTH!

Should I sterilize her water? It is not necessary to boil the water you give to your baby to drink either by bottle or cup, or that you use to mix formula. As long as it is properly treated, you may use the tap water in your home that is supplied by your town. If you have a well, be certain that it is shocked and tested as safe to drink. If you purchase and use bottled water, avoid the use of water that has had fluoride added to it.

Spit Happens

The spitty baby may have gastroesophageal (GE) reflux. This is a mechanical phenomenon common to most babies. All babies probably have a bit of reflux, but most do not have any symptom from it. With symptomatic reflux, babies usually spit up within thirty minutes following a feeding. A portion of the feeding returns up the esophagus and out of the mouth. GE reflux is generally outgrown by one year of life, often sooner. There is treatment available for your baby.

Reflux is common and usually not significant. In rare cases, babies lose enough of their feedings so as not to gain sufficient weight. If your pediatrician suspects that the baby has reflux, he or she may recommend treatment. Rest assured that the therapies used for this are not harmful. First, elevation of the head is helpful; gravity helps. Keep your baby at an angle, unless she is supine for a diaper change. Thickening feeds with cereal may be advised. Of course, this only works with bottle-feeding. A medication such as ranitidine may be used, but only if needed.

HEADS UP

When you bring your newborn home, consider elevating the crib mattress slightly so as to have her head elevated all of the time, except when changing her. This slight angle will allow gravity to keep her feedings in the stomach, rather than the temptation to ride up the esophagus toward the throat. This helps to prevent gastroesophageal reflux. It is both comfy and helpful to keep them with their "heads up!"

Postpartum Blues

Postpartum blues—do they really exist? They really do. Some women are affected by them, and some women are completely untouched. They can occur anytime in the first year after giving birth, but they usually happen within the first four weeks. The blues can arise unexpectedly in the midst of the joy of your new baby, creating confusion as to why. It may be quite frustrating for you.

Generally thought to be due in large part to the changes in your hormone levels, there are many factors that can lead to the blues. Yes, they are probably hormonally induced, as are the expected mood changes that happen during pregnancy and following the birth of a baby. Added to the hormonal flux are your fatigue, anxiety over newborn care, and perhaps feelings of being overwhelmed by the changes taking place in your life. You are now responsible for another life, and this has filled your plate greatly.

33

Be reassured that you are not alone. More than half of women experience the blues to some degree. They usually last no more than two weeks. If the blues increase or last more than two weeks, you may have postpartum depression. Real depression only affects a small percentage of women.

Postpartum blues can include intermittent and unexpected feelings of sadness, tearfulness, and crying. Real depression can also occur and must be treated seriously. Depression may be more likely if you have any history of mental health concerns, such as anxiety or depression, no matter how mild. It also is more apt to happen if you have been affected by stressors during your pregnancy, such as moving to a new home, suffering the loss of a loved one, financial concerns, or a rocky relationship with your partner, friends, or co-workers.

Acknowledge Your Feelings

If you are having any unanticipated feelings, always be honest. You have done nothing wrong, and there is nothing wrong with you. This may be totally unexpected by you. It really is out of the blue. Try to get as much rest as possible. This will help lessen the postpartum blues. Rest when your baby rests. Try to lessen the stressors in your life if possible. Enlist your family members to do the same on your behalf.

Share your feelings openly with your partner. Remember that you endured the pregnancy and delivered a baby. Your family and friends should be there for you, willing and able to give you the support that you need at this time.

As your life changes, plan to share responsibilities in new ways, such as sharing chores, grocery shopping, and baby care at home. The caring and compassionate partner will step up to the plate for you. He knows that you have to be healthy for the baby to remain healthy.

Ask for Help

If the postpartum blues are any more than mild and brief, know your limits and speak up. Signs of worsening include difficulty concentrating, negative feelings toward your baby, insomnia, decreased appetite, less energy, agitation, and unhappiness.

Do not hesitate to alert your partner that you need help. There is wonderful help for postpartum depression today. Ask your obstetrician or your pediatrician for a referral to a qualified psychiatrist. Therapy is available, including short-term medication use when needed.

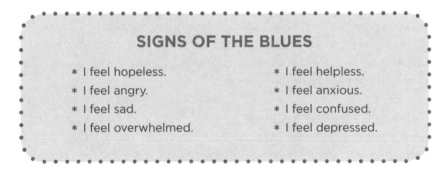

SIGNS OF THE BLUES

* I feel hopeless.
* I feel angry.
* I feel sad.
* I feel overwhelmed.

* I feel helpless.
* I feel anxious.
* I feel confused.
* I feel depressed.

CHAPTER FOUR

The First Doctor Visit

It's time to visit the pediatrician for the first time at the office! Now that your baby is out of the hospital and safely home, you must be tired after the first night. It's important to bring your little one in the next day to check on her weight and color and to ask any questions that you may have. If this is your first child, everything is new to you, and it can be overwhelming.

The first visit serves many purposes. Newborns can be discharged from the hospital after only two days, depending on when you deliver and the route by which you delivered the baby. It's imperative that we monitor the weight and color of your baby right away. We wish to make certain that feedings are going well for both of you, and that weight loss has not exceeded the amount expected. Also, the baby's skin color may be jaundiced, with a yellow or orange hue, and that should be checked as well. The peak bilirubin level in the baby's bloodstream is generally at three days of life, which is what causes the jaundice that is visible on their skin. We don't want that to go unnoticed if it is slowly increasing beyond what is expected.

Your pediatrician will examine your baby briefly, check his weight, and examine his skin color carefully. The weight will be taken unclothed, as it was in the hospital nursery, so that it will be as consistent as possible. Always support the head and neck and the bottom as you lift, hold, and transfer to the scale. Do not worry about specific numbers. They may be slightly off due to different scales. Large discrepancies are the main concern, and these are uncommon and usually related to feeding difficulties. So enjoy the first visit for the weight and color check, and be certain to jot down your questions. You may be a bit too tired to recall them!

Exam Time

The first exam in the office takes place directly following discharge from the hospital. Your baby is weighed and examined closely for jaundice. Each examination that follows takes place at routinely scheduled visits called "health care maintenance" visits. They are also known as well-baby visits. During these visits your baby is again weighed on the scale with her diaper off (briefly!), and measurements for growth are performed. These include the baby's weight, length, and head circumference. Once these are completed, usually by the pediatric nurse, your pediatrician will perform a complete head-to-toe examination. He will examine every part of the baby's body carefully.

Starting with the head, he will examine the baby's skull and scalp for any abnormalities. He will check the anterior fontanel ("soft spot" on top of the skull). The face is next to be checked, including the eyes, ears, nose, mouth, and throat. He will check for the neck to be supple. The chest exam includes listening to the breath sounds and the heart sounds. When the abdomen is palpated, the doctor is evaluating the organs that live within. He will also check out the umbilical cord site for healing. The arms and legs are evaluated for strength, reflexes, and any deformities. Your baby's skin will also be scrutinized for any birthmarks that may not have been evident earlier.

Plumbing parts are special and need special care. Boys tend to be easier. Simply lift the boy's scrotum and wipe everything. Don't forget the groin creases. Boys aim, so be careful! Always wipe front to back for girls, or top to bottom. Wipe downward gently through her sensitive midline structures. Once weekly, you may clean the groove between the large labia and the small labia on each side. Simply use a moistened Q-tip with soft downward strokes to clean the cream and/or stool that can collect there.

On the Scale

Prior to the examination at each well visit, your baby will be weighed and measured. This allows for consistent monitoring of growth over time. There are logs throughout this book so that you too can keep track of your baby's growth over time and have a record to refer to if you have any questions about your baby's health in the future. Weights and lengths will be done with the diaper off for pure measurements. Please move back while your baby boy is being weighed. You may be hit by a steady stream of urine!

Follow that Curve

Growth curves are useful tools to confirm consistent growth over time.

Some pediatricians measure the circumference of your baby's chest. Some will not, and that is fine. All pediatricians will follow weight, length, and head circumference. The full exam will be reported to you, and any new findings will be discussed.

| 37

The Soft Spot

The doctor will examine the anterior fontanel on the top of the skull. This is the "soft spot" where the bones of the skull have not yet come together. The space fibroses, fills, and fuses, usually by eighteen months of age. The anterior fontanel space can be seen to pulsate, and this is normal. Don't be afraid to touch it. It won't bother your baby.

Growth

Every baby is unique and different. Some are born large, and some are born small. Some have medical issues that contribute to their size, but most do not. This is what makes the world go round! Some parents are overly concerned with growth when they need not be. Some uncommon

NOTEABLES

Date: _____

Age: _____

Weight: _____

Length: _____

Head Circumference: _____

Notes from Visit: _____

_____

_____

_____

_____

_____

_____

_____

_____

medical entities can lead to certain birth weights. For example, a smaller baby is expected with prematurity, maternal smoking, and IUGR (intra-uterine growth retardation). A larger baby can be a result of maternal diabetes, gestational or otherwise. Your obstetrician will be monitoring your pregnancy for any of these uncommon complications. When babies are born without any medical issues, they do just fine despite their size. Ironically, smaller babies are often more feisty!

Don't be so concerned with your baby's birth weight and birth length, or with her measurements at each well visit in the office. Rather, be pleased to hear from your pediatrician that all is well with your baby's examination, and that her growth is consistent over time (no matter the percentile) and well proportioned. As long as this is the case, growth is normal. Some of us are small, some are medium, and some are large. Bigger isn't always better! Your baby is fine just the way she is.

Pediatricians are often asked about percentiles. Parents may hear friends or relatives speak of their child's grand height and weight percentiles, and then everyone is led to compare and fret. Although size is not exclusively a concern for dads, many do ask if their son will be big enough to play on the line on a football team, or be big and strong enough to hit a grand slam. Truly, the only concern for you and the pediatrician is that your baby's growth is consistent over time and well proportioned.

A Head Above the Rest

Your baby's head circumference will be measured at each well visit through eighteen months of age. The anterior fontanel is usually closed by that time. All of the sutures of the skull should be fused by then. The head circumference measurement is regarded by many to be the most important measurement to follow. It represents not only the growth of the bones of the skull, but also of the developing brain.

Development

At every well-baby appointment, your pediatrician will spend time assessing the baby's developmental status—an important part of every checkup. She will ask questions that pertain to the things you have observed your baby doing. The combination of your answers and the doctor's observations during her examination will lead to the analysis of your baby's developmental status.

The range of normal is wide, so don't be alarmed. For example, first steps alone can occur anywhere between nine months and eighteen months of age. Most will walk at around thirteen months. Another example is the first words used in context. Most will have three words that are used in context by fifteen months of age. Some infants use this many words before their first birthday, but some wait beyond fifteen months, particularly if a sibling is doing a good bit of talking for them!

Don't compare to others, especially to your first child. Despite the same gene pool, siblings can differ greatly. Also, remember that medical issues can alter the achievement of milestones. Chronic middle ear fluid, with or without ear infections, can delay the development of expressive language. The fluid is a barrier, and the infant hears as if she is underwater; hence, speech is delayed. Always rely on the doctor to guide you regarding your baby's developmental progress.

Development encompasses several areas of progressive activity. Motor development is both gross motor and fine motor. Gross motor applies to the roll, scoot, creep, crawl, pull-to-stand, cruise, and walk progression. Fine motor applies to what babies do with their hands, such as transferring objects, using the pincer grasp, and self-feeding. Speech/language development is both receptive and expressive. Receptive speech includes hearing and processing, and expressive speech applies to what a baby says and when he says it. Social development has to do with relatedness and your baby's reaction to his environment over time. Watch all of this development along with your pediatrician.

Are We Connected?

One of the most important features of normal development is the feeling of connection with your baby. He will respond to your calm, gentle ways.

If you don't feel this connection, be certain to discuss this with your pediatrician. Medical issues such as colic can delay connection. Never fear . . . once medical issues have resolved, your bond and connection will be as wonderful as ever! Your baby knows that you have been there with him since day one, caring for him each day.

Watch Together

Observe your baby independently and with your partner. Read about developmental milestones, but don't rely on specific numbers, ages, dates, and goals to the letter. Remember that your baby is unique and special. If she is out of the normal range for a given part of her development, your pediatrician will alert you.

Watch Me Grow and Change

At each well-baby visit, developmental progress is reviewed. Your pediatrician will ask you many questions that pertain to your baby's developmental progress. The answers you give will help the doctor determine whether or not there is a developmental delay. If a delay is suspected, your pediatrician will recommend an evaluation. Early intervention is the best intervention.

Feeding

You have a beautiful baby to care for, and that means feeding him. As you know, newborns require frequent feedings. By the end of the first year of life, they will even enjoy routine mealtimes with the family! So hang in there; this will get easier. The responsibility resides with parents and chosen caretakers to feed a baby adequately. You will be guided by friends and relatives on this subject, but rely primarily on the advice of your pediatrician, her staff, and her literature.

By four to six months of age, you will begin to give your baby solids by spoon, but until that time he will have a liquid diet. Whether you are breast-feeding or formula-feeding, begin with a schedule in mind. Initial feedings should be given on demand, but the usual recommendation is every three hours by day and only on demand through the night. Breast-fed babies will increase their time at the breast as their age, weight, and energy increase, and they will work up to a time of active suckling of fifteen to twenty minutes per side. Formula-fed babies will begin taking one to two ounces, and they will also increase this volume as they and their needs grow. As time passes, solids will be introduced. Your pediatrician's obligation to you is to lead you through the appropriate feeding of your baby during this vital first year and beyond.

Pediatricians recommend and support breast-feeding as optimal nutrition for new babies. There is a culture of disdain today for those who decide not to breast-feed. This is quite unfair. Sometimes breast-feeding fails, and there may be many contributing factors: medical, emotional, or physical. Sometimes breast-feeding is simply not chosen. You must not feel any guilt in this regard. Family, friends, and society should support you no matter what. Formula-fed babies receive adequate nutrition, and you can bond just as well with your baby.

Breast-Feeding

Breast-feeding is an art, not a science. There are no set rules. Try to relax. Your baby will sense any stress. Stay calm to stay successful. A supportive nursing bra will be very helpful to you. Also make sure that you have enough support below the arm holding your baby. Breast milk is thinner than formula, but no less rich. It is full of the calories and nutrients your baby needs.

Bottle-Feeding

Formula-feeding is an acceptable alternative to breast-feeding. The formula you use should be iron-fortified and prepared carefully according to the directions. Sterilization of bottles and nipples is unnecessary. Wash these as you would the dishes in the sink or in the dishwasher. Formula is available as ready-to-feed, powder, and liquid concentrate. If your baby shows an intolerance to a particular formula, your pediatrician may advise a change to a different formula. This is uncommon. The incidence may be a bit higher if there is a family history of a food allergy or sensitivity.

| 43

Take it Easy

If you are using expressed breast milk or are formula-feeding, allow loved ones to help you so that you may rest on occasion. If siblings are old enough and well supervised, they can carefully help to feed your baby too.

EBM, or expressed breast milk, may be used within three to four days if properly refrigerated. It may be frozen and stored for use within three months. Dads and others love to bond with feedings, either with EBM or formula, both of which are delivered by bottle. By all means, let those around you help!

Breast and Bottle

If you are breast-feeding, your pediatrician may suggest supplementing with a triple vitamin (A, D, and C). Most medications come through your milk, and most will not harm the baby. Call your pediatrician to be certain that you can safely feed your baby if you need to take medication. Formula-fed babies do not require vitamin supplementation. Bottled or boiled water is not necessary to mix powdered or concentrated formula. Properly shocked and tested well water or public town water will suffice.

Hot Shots

Vaccination against life-threatening infections will keep your baby safe. Prevention is indeed the best cure. With the help of your pediatrician, your job as a parent is to prevent suffering of any kind in your children. With vaccination against significant viral and bacterial infections, we have the opportunity to prevent suffering and perhaps even death. Many infections can be life threatening in the first two years of life. Thankfully, your baby has many antibodies from your immune system transferred through the placenta. These provide protection only from the diseases to which you are immune. They are wonderful protection for your baby initially, but they dwindle by four to six months of life. Thereafter, your baby must build her own immune system, with vaccines and with each illness she may contract.

A great amount of study over many years by many experts in the field of infectious disease has resulted in today's recommended immunization schedule. Over time, vaccines have become safer and more effective for your baby. The first vaccine may be given in the newborn nursery at the hospital, or it may be given within two weeks at the pediatric office. With the guidance of your pediatrician, your baby should receive vaccines at each well baby visit during her first two years. This will complete the initial series of recommended vaccinations. At some visits, several vaccinations may be given, and this is safe to do. Adverse reactions to vaccinations are uncommon today and are usually confined to low-grade temperature elevation, fussiness, or local redness and swelling. If these occur, they are temporary and harmless to your baby.

Not that many years ago, thousands suffered and many died from diseases that have significantly decreased in number. For example, smallpox took many lives before it was eradicated by vaccine. We must not let our guard down. If we fail to vaccinate, infectious disease will return to our children with a vengeance.

Here it Comes

Vaccines are given intramuscularly. The skin is cleansed with alcohol prior to the administration. The syringe is held at an angle so that the muscle is reached with the injection. The anterior (front) part of the thigh is used through six months of age.

From nine months of age onward, the deltoid muscle (shoulder) may be used. Your baby will feel the injection, and she will probably cry, but just briefly, since you will immediately hold her and console her.

What's in the Vial?

Vaccines contain antigens from specific diseases. They are in small quantity or are weakened. Prior to 2001, multidose vials of vaccine contained the preservative thiomersal to prevent bacteria and fungi from contaminating each vial.

Thiomersal accumulation from many vaccines led to increased levels of ethylmercury, which may affect child development. Since 2001, vaccines given to children have been single-dose vaccinations that are virtually preservative-free. The vaccines are used in a timely fashion so as not to require the use of the preservative.

Family Affair

Moral support from your partner is helpful when your baby receives vaccinations. Shots can hurt mom more than they hurt baby. The AAP, FDA, and the CDC work very hard to ensure the safety of all of the vaccines recommended for your baby. After much valid scientific study, there is no evidence to associate vaccines with developmental entities such as autism.

Your pediatrician will advise vaccination at each well-baby visit according to the current recommendations.

AT EVERY CHECKUP

Your pediatrician will cover certain areas of growth and development at each well-baby visit, beginning with the complete physical examination.

* She will review your baby's growth velocity since the last visit, referring to standard growth charts. Follow that curve!
* She will also assess and review developmental progress and let you know what gains to expect by the next visit.
* Finally, your baby's doctor will discuss vitamins, vaccines, lab tests, feeding, or referrals as pertains to age, in addition to answering any of your questions.

CHAPTER FIVE

Two-Week Wellness Visit

It is time to see the pediatrician for the first well-baby visit! Health care maintenance—this is the real name for the well-baby visit or routine checkup. How exciting . . . this is your baby's first one! You have survived the first two weeks, and by now you must be tired. Your baby is probably still confused between night and day. Now it's time for you to sit down, rest, and make certain that your baby is doing well in all ways.

Remember to bring the diaper bag with you whenever you travel with your baby. If you forget supplies, don't be worried. The pediatric office will have supplies that you can use if needed. Drive safely, and if you need assistance ask freely. It's helpful to have your partner accompany you to this first visit, because you can use the help and you won't need to repeat all that you have learned.

You will be asked how everyone is faring since delivery and since you have been at home. Be honest and accurate so that the staff can record everything in the chart. They want to hear the good, the bad, and the ugly!

The pediatric nurse will ask you to undress the baby down to the diaper in order to get precise measurements. When you are finished, the length, weight, and head circumference will be measured by the pediatric nurse and recorded in your baby's medical record, though the head circumference may be measured by the doctor. The interim history and measurements may be recorded in either a paper chart or in an electronic medical record using a computer. Your pediatrician will be referring to this record after the examination is completed. After the nurse has completed her time with you, the pediatrician will come in and greet you both. He may ask some of the same questions, so bear with him.

Exam Time

Hold the baby in your arms until the doctor arrives to do the examination. If there is a wait, use the time to review the questions that you may have for him during your visit. The pediatrician will examine your baby from head to toe, with you right beside him. He or she will examine the baby gently yet thoroughly, evaluating every part of the body.

You will be close enough to observe the doctor as he looks at every part of your baby's body. He will most likely speak as he goes, pointing out any nuances that are of note during the examination. The pediatrician will also be watching for signs of normal early development while he is performing the examination.

He may ask you questions during the exam time, and you should feel free to ask questions at this time as well.

Beginning with the head, he will examine the skull, scalp, and the anterior fontanel. He will look at facial features, and he will examine the baby's eyes, ears, nose, mouth, and throat. Next, he will listen to the heart and lungs with the stethoscope. Then he will gently palpate the abdomen, inspect the genitalia, and then examine the extremities for muscle tone, pulses, and reflexes. Voilà! Your baby has just been fully examined from head to tiny little toe!

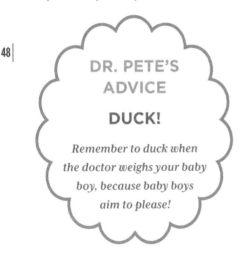

DR. PETE'S ADVICE

DUCK!

Remember to duck when the doctor weighs your baby boy, because baby boys aim to please!

48

NOTEABLES

Date: _____

Age: _____

Weight: _____

Length: _____

Head Circumference: _____

Notes from Visit: _____

_____

_____

_____

_____

_____

_____

_____

_____

_____

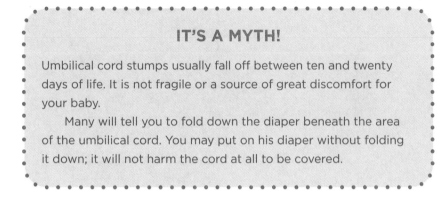

IT'S A MYTH!

Umbilical cord stumps usually fall off between ten and twenty days of life. It is not fragile or a source of great discomfort for your baby.

Many will tell you to fold down the diaper beneath the area of the umbilical cord. You may put on his diaper without folding it down; it will not harm the cord at all to be covered.

Growth and Development

At two weeks of age, most babies regain—if not exceed—their birth weight. This should occur as long as feeding is successful. There is no set formula for the increases in her growth, but your pediatrician will let you know if the gains are sufficient. Again, remember that percentiles are not as important as consistent growth over time.

By now your baby should have increased in length by at least half an inch. Her head circumference should have increased as well. Her head may look large and out of proportion with her weight and length, and this is normal for many babies. With time, her body will catch up to the size of her head! In rare circumstances the head is too large, which is a condition called macrocephaly. Conversely, microcephaly refers to a head that is too small. This is also rare, and the doctor will review this if it exists.

As far as developmental progress is concerned, babies begin to do more than just feed and sleep. At each well visit, the doctor will ask questions and also observe your baby to assess appropriate development. Always consider motor, speech, intellectual, and social development.

At this age, she should be moving her arms and legs symmetrically, have a great grip with each hand, and follow you with her eyes as you move slowly in front of her. Reflexes should be normal. Vocalization includes cooing in addition to crying. She will respond to sounds with a startle, a cry, or a blink. You will notice that your baby has a bit more wakeful time, and she will be unhappy if over- or understimulated. She will be soothed by your voice and your touch, and she can make eye contact at close range. She may grin, but this is usually due to either gas or milk bliss!

Baby's Behavior

Normal newborn behaviors are still present at two weeks of age, including sneezing, eye crossing, and periodic breathing. Sneezing and hiccups can be present for the first two months of life, and no treatment is needed. Your baby may respond instantly to different sounds. She may blink, cry, startle, or become quiet depending on the sound. Enjoy the changes in your baby, as each day brings something new and exciting to see.

|51

How Reflexive

Most behavior is reflexive at this age. In addition to reflexive behavior, neurologic reflexes should be present. The Moro, or startle reflex, can occur in response to touch or sound, or without any stimulation at all.

Your baby's arms will rise abruptly, her hands will open with fingers extended, and her lips may quiver. Within seconds she will calm and be relaxed again. This normal neurologic reflex may last for two to three months.

Get a Grip

You may be surprised at the strength and quality of your baby's grip, which is also reflexive and quite normal. Her hands may seem flexed or clenched much of the time. This is also expected. She will inadvertently reach up and scratch her face.

Arms and legs should move up and down symmetrically as you move her, but not necessarily with purpose. Always support your baby's head, as she is unable to do so herself as yet. Her head will seem floppy to you, but it is normal.

Let's Communicate

Your two-week-old baby is already communicating with you in many ways. Her phonation is there for the listening. She makes ooh and ah sounds, and she coos actively. Your baby will cry to be held, changed, or fed. She may cry if over- or understimulated. She will yawn and sigh, and she will especially enjoy eye contact with you. She will be calmed by the sound of your voice.

Feeding

A regular routine will set the stage for a reasonable daily feeding pattern. Hopefully by now you and your baby have settled into a reasonable feeding schedule. You probably no longer have to wake him every three hours for feedings during the day. He should wake up on his own. Also, he is most likely stretching out the feeding intervals at night. By now the breast-fed two-week-old should be content for at least two, if not three, hours following a full feeding with your milk. The formula-fed baby will advance his volume of feeding as he grows, with a different number of ounces for each infant. He may be taking two to three ounces per feeding at this point. You may judge any baby's fullness by the number of hours he remains content before demanding the next feeding.

Remember that you may allow yourself to take a break. Feeding your baby is time-intensive, wonderful work, but it is hard work. You may not need a break, but consider your partner or another trusted friend or family member to give an occasional feeding for you. They will certainly enjoy doing this for you, and you can enjoy some much-needed rest. Remember that you must be happy and healthy for your baby to be happy and healthy! Dads look forward to giving an evening feeding after returning from work.

If you are breast-feeding, you can use that time to express milk. This serves two purposes: It relieves you of your milk for comfort, and it builds your supply of stored EBM.

EBM, or expressed breast milk, is commonly used for infants under many different circumstances. It can be given to preterm babies who need to be cared for in the neonatal intensive care unit, and it can be given if you require medication that should not be transferred to your baby. In this case, you will temporarily be advised to "pump and dump."

Breast-Feeding

Your breast milk is rich in calories and nutrients and is the ideal nutrition for your newborn baby. Find the position that is most comfortable for you, keeping your baby at a slightly elevated angle. Stay relaxed while feeding. You can nurse your baby anywhere as long as you are covered and comfortable doing so. One distinct advantage of breast-feeding is that there is nothing to forget at home!

Breast Pumps for EBM

There are a variety of breast pumps available to you for expressing your breast milk, and there are many reasons to pump. You can use a manual, battery-powered, or electric breast pump. They may be single- or double-pumping. You may find the electric pump to be more efficient, and the double pump will take the least time. Breast pumps are helpful to relieve engorgement, to reverse inverted nipples, and to maintain or increase your milk supply.

Bottle-Feeding

Formula is an acceptable alternative to breast milk. It is also rich in calories and nutrients. Please don't add cereal to the bottle, unless instructed to do so by your pediatrician (as in the case of a baby with reflux). You must remember to bring the formula and preparation materials with you when you are away from home. Most two-week-old babies will take between two and three ounces per feeding.

Formula Preparation

When preparing formula, you must be careful to follow the mixing instructions. Powdered and liquid concentrate must be mixed with water. It does not need to be boiled water. Tap will do. Formula may be given at room temperature. Your baby will probably reject cold formula, but it need not be warm. The FDA oversees manufacturers of infant formulas to ensure that they comply with their nutritional and safety requirements.

Hot Shots

At each well visit, your baby's pediatrician will advise you on vaccinating according to current recommendations. Vaccine protocols are agreed upon by many agencies after many studies and medical research. Many newborns receive their first vaccination in the newborn nursery. They are not too young to receive this. If your baby did not receive his first vaccination in the hospital, he will receive it at the two-week checkup. This will probably traumatize you more than him. The tissues in the exam room are really for mommy's tears!

The recommended vaccination at this age is the hepatitis B vaccine. Hepatitis is a viral infection that affects the entire body, but primarily causes liver inflammation. If one contracts hepatitis, and if it causes liver failure, there is no definitive treatment or cure. Liver transplants do not work. Although liver failure is rare, it is so important to protect your children from this infection. Hepatitis B is contracted via exposure to blood or intimate secretions.

You may think your baby is not at all at risk for this type of hepatitis in infancy, and you are correct, unless he is exposed to the blood of someone with this form of hepatitis. Although the risk of exposure is low for most infants and children, administration of the vaccination for hepatitis B is recommended in the first days or weeks of life. Research has proven the vaccine to be safe when administered to newborns and young infants, and there are three vaccines in the series. Your baby will receive all three of the hepatitis B vaccines before her first birthday.

Your baby's vaccine will be prepared by carefully drawing it into a syringe using aseptic techniques. This vaccine is a single-dose vaccine, one dose per vial, and it does not contain any preservative. The vaccine will be drawn up either by the pediatric nurse or by your pediatrician. Vaccines should be given by a qualified and licensed nurse, not by a medical assistant or receptionist.

Vaccinations are administered intramuscularly—that is, directly into your baby's muscle. Prior to any injection, the skin at the site is prepped with alcohol, usually with a small alcohol prep pad. This cleanses the intended site of the injection so as to prevent any subsequent skin infection. It is possible to have an infection at the site because the skin has been compromised by a needle, but this is rare indeed. If infection occurs, the site will show signs of redness, swelling, possible discharge, and tenderness to the touch. The injection is administered quickly and efficiently in order for discomfort to be minimized. The anterior thigh is the usual location for the injection through at least six months of age. Most babies do cry when they receive vaccines, but they calm down within minutes.

Once your baby has received his vaccination, pick him up immediately to console him in your arms. Rock him as you walk or sway, and speak softly to him with reassurance, even at this young age. Most injection sites don't bleed afterward, but some may. It is rare to have a bleeding dyscrasia that affects clotting. If there is a drop of blood, the site will be blotted with gauze and a Band-Aid will be applied. Subsequent skin infection is rarely seen.

See the chapter 12 for a special Immunization Record where you can log your baby's vaccines.

What's Next?

After the measurements, examination, and vaccinations, your pediatrician will review your baby's overall health and development, and she will prepare you for the coming months. This part of the visit comprises all of the information you need to understand how your baby's ongoing health is monitored, both for you and with you. Parents and pediatricians are integral members of the team that helps to raise a child. As such, much is reviewed before your visit can be called complete. We are in this together!

At the two-week checkup, your pediatrician explained any new findings from your baby's examination. Perhaps she had a blocked tear duct. Blocked tear ducts, or dacryostenosis, are common, usually in one eye but sometimes in both. Your pediatrician will instruct you on the proper way to massage the tear duct in order to help it resolve. Massaging twice daily is the ticket to resolution, and secondary infection is uncommon. Place your clean finger next to your baby's nose, under the corner of the eye. That's where the lacrimal duct runs vertically. Gently massage the area back and forth, up and down for thirty to sixty seconds twice daily. If colorful eye discharge appears, call your pediatrician for an appointment.

You most likely received a normal result from the state newborn screening, which includes testing for concerns such as phenylketonuria, galactosemia, hypothyroidism, HIV, enzyme defects, and inborn errors of metabolism, among others. These are entities that otherwise may go undetected. The newborn screen is a wonderful tool used in hospitals during the first days of life. A sample of blood is taken from your baby's heel and is then sent to your state department of health. This state screening tests for many significant medical maladies that are not apparent on physical examination. Your pediatrician should have received the results of the newborn screen by this time, and they will be discussed. If you receive a borderline result, the test must be repeated immediately. A positive result is rare.

During the two-week checkup, you were also able to review the features of your baby's stool. You will soon become a connoisseur. Remember that each infant is unique, and they may have different stool patterns. Consistency is more important than frequency of stool, and one pediatrician has said that anything between marbles and white wine is fine! Whatever the issue at hand, your pediatrician is committed to explaining everything to you in terms that are understandable.

DR. PETE'S ADVICE

CONNOISSEUR OF CACA

* *Newborn stool varies widely depending on the individual baby and the type of feeding he receives.*
* *Breast-fed babies usually have loose, seedy, mustard-colored stool. Formula-fed babies usually have pastier, darker stool.*
* *Consistency of stool is important. Frequency is not. Some babies go twelve times daily, and some go one to two times per week.*
* *Diarrheal stool in infancy is like colored water. Constipated stool in infancy is small and pellet-like.*

DERMA DILEMMA!

If cradle cap appears on the scalp, you will be told what to do. Your baby's skin is sensitive. Some babies are more sensitive than others, and sensitivity can be a familial trait. Cradle cap is seborrheic dermatitis on the scalp. It is an inflammation that causes yellow-colored scales on the skin. If the case is mild, it does not cause itchiness or pain. It is certainly not contagious, nor is it necessarily a harbinger of eczema. Your doctor will recommend a medicated shampoo to apply by gently massaging with a soft brush every other day. In some cultures the scalp is covered with olive oil and cradle cap scales are lifted off gently with a comb. This does no harm, but it can be quite messy, and your baby may smell like a salad!

Final Questions

Are there more issues to review before you have completed this first well-baby appointment? We are not quite done yet! The physical growth of your baby is very important and will be monitored closely for you. Your pediatrician will review growth with you at each well-baby visit, including weight, length, and head circumference. He will chart the measurements and share the growth curves with you to see your baby's progress. You should have seen the growth chart for your baby, with plots for birth measurements, as well as plots for the measurements taken at the weight check at two to four days of life. Now the two-week measurements have been plotted, and the growth velocity should be consistent, as long as feedings have been successful and well tolerated by the baby. The head circumference may seem more generous compared to his or her weight and length, and this is normal. The body size will catch up to the head size with time. Remember that percentiles are not as important as consistent growth velocity over time.

Your baby probably received the hepatitis B vaccine, or HBV, which carries no history of significant adverse effects. On a rare occasion, an infant may have a small local reaction at the site of the injection, including slight redness or swelling. If it seems tender to touch, you may use a warm compress for soothing. It is best not to use any pain reliever for this. Most pediatricians advise against the use of analgesics in the first two months of life, as it could mask the signs of serious infection in your baby.

Your first full well-baby visit is nearing completion, and your questions are being answered. Your baby is well, and your pediatrician will be reassuring you of all the aspects of this visit that are normal. The doctor will also apprise you of any issue that is of concern regarding your baby's health at this time. Do not worry . . . if there is a concern, your doctor will explain it fully and go over the plan to address it.

Now it is time to leave the pediatric office. This concludes the first official visit for your baby's health care maintenance. Be sure that your

QUESTIONS TO ASK

Now is the time to ask any questions that have not already been answered by the doctor:

* Is my baby's exam totally normal?
* Is she developmentally age-appropriate?
* Is she growing well?
* Does she need any medication?
* Are there any adverse effects to look for from the vaccine?
* Will her hair ever grow?
* Will she ever sleep through the night?

questions are answered fully before leaving. If you think of something later, simply call the office. Be certain that you have all that you came with. With so much to think about, new mothers often overlook a belonging or two. You should have your purse, your keys, the diaper bag, any literature or prescriptions, and of course your baby! Don't go home without her!

Looking Ahead

The next developmental milestones should occur by the next well visit, which is at two months of age. Watch for the baby to follow more with her eyes, to see farther, and to develop a social smile. She will be babbling even more, and she should have more wakeful daytime hours. Be certain to ask all of your questions before leaving, and continue to enjoy your lovely two-week-old baby! Keep up the good work, and get enough rest! You are doing a great job!

CHAPTER SIX

Two-Month Wellness Visit

It is now time to return to the pediatric office for the two-month well-baby appointment. Six weeks have passed since the last well visit. Think of all the things you have to report. Dress your baby comfortably, according to the season, and be certain not to overdress her. You may have to adjust the straps in the car seat, as her size has changed significantly by this time.

Here you are at the pediatric office again, and this time you are toting a carrier that is much heavier than it was before. You are building your biceps! At the office waiting room, sit away from coughing children if possible. Most waiting rooms don't separate well and ill patients. Once in the examination room, undress your baby for the examination. Your baby may be chilly during the exam, but don't worry as this is less troubling at this age. Hold her for warmth and comfort. She may not enjoy the examination today because she has begun to be more aware of her surroundings. She will be looking about the room, now able to fix and focus at greater distance.

Once the doctor comes in, he will greet you both and then begin the two-month examination. After your baby is weighed and measured, it's time for her to be fully examined. Much has changed by now, and this will be evident to you. She will regard the doctor as she is examined, and she may not be pleased to be naked on the exam table. Crying is expected during this exam. Your baby is not in pain . . . she is feeling vulnerable. At this age, she is soothed by faces that she knows. She has not seen her doctor that often. If possible, allow her to see your face during the examination.

Exam Time

Your pediatrician will gently perform the examination from head to toe, pointing out any findings. Most pediatricians will explain any findings as they appear so that you can see them and understand. Let's start from the top as usual. First, the scalp and hair (if there is any) are checked, and the anterior fontanel is palpated. This is still open on top of her head, and it will feel full when your baby is supine. This is normal. The baby's skin will be inspected from head to toe as the exam progresses. Her eyes, ears, nose, mouth, and throat will be thoroughly checked. Her neck is then examined for any lumps and bumps and is tested for suppleness. The chest is listened to for heart sounds, which should be normal and without a heart murmur. Your pediatrician will then listen to her breath sounds as well, which should be nice and clear. Palpating the abdomen is next, finding a soft, non-tender belly with normal-size organs within. He will inspect the genitalia to ensure that the structures are normal, with appropriate growth. The extremities are tested for strength, muscle tone, reflexes, and hip dysplasia.

In addition, your baby's neurologic status is evaluated with observation and examination. When two-month-old infants are neurologically intact, they have age-appropriate development as well as normal physical findings, including normal muscle tone and various normal reflexes. Your pediatrician may lift your baby to test overall tone in the horizontal position. The examination is complete, but be certain to ask any questions about her body before she is dressed again.

Growth and Development

At two months of age, your baby's physical growth may surprise you. Infants will usually gain one to one and a half inches per month during this time. Their head circumference may increase by one half inch per month, and they will have gained some pounds and ounces.

NOTEABLES

Date: _____

Age: _____

Weight: _____

Length: _____

Head Circumference: _____

Notes from Visit: _____

_____

_____

_____

_____

_____

_____

_____

_____

_____

_____

DR. PETE'S ADVICE

WHAT A PAIN

Medication has probably not been advised for your baby during the first two months of his life. It is now safe to administer medication, but you are restricted to but a few different medications. You may give simethicone for colic, ranitidine for reflux, and acetaminophen for pain relief if medically indicated. Always remember that medication should only be used if absolutely necessary, and your pediatrician will give you the appropriate dosage based on your baby's weight

In terms of development, there is so much more to see now, especially in the areas of motor, speech, intellect, and social development. Your little one should now be following, or tracking visually side to side. He can temporarily lift his head while pressing up with his arms when he is prone during tummy time. He may be more relaxed, less twitchy, and his hands will be open more often than before. He will have an awesome grip. Babble will increase as you see his personality begin to emerge. With more new sounds, you will see that he can now display different emotions.

Intellectually, your baby has become more aware of his surroundings and more responsive to you and your emotions as well. He will calm to your voice as always and should be easily comforted when crying. You will also be able to discern the needs that he wants met by the cry that he gives. He may begin to play with his fingers, and they will often be found in his mouth, accompanied by copious drooling. This is an early sign of teething, although you will probably not see teeth for many more months.

Finally, the social interaction that you have at this age will melt your heart. Your baby should be responsive to your touch, your voice, and your face as he responds with that lovely social smile. This smile is a direct response to you and to the loving care that he has received from you, his mother.

DERMA DILEMMA: YEAST DERMATITIS

Yeast infections are common fungal infections that can affect the mucous membranes of the mouth as well as the skin. Yeast growth occurs in warm, moist areas—which, by definition, a diaper is! Also when broad spectrum antibiotics are needed for a bacterial infection, all bacterial flora are reduced, leading to an overgrowth of yeast. The treatment of choice for a yeast infection, or monilial dermatitis, is topical antifungal cream.

Baby's Behavior

At two months of age, your baby has become much more aware of the world around her. Your pediatrician will closely observe her reactions during the examination, and he will test the baby's tone with a horizontal lift.

Two-month-olds will relax their clenched fists and suck on their fingers quite often, which is an early sign of teething. Your baby will now have more strength in her head and neck, but she still cannot do without your support there.

Get a Grip!

Your two-month-old can still grip fiercely, and he may try to lift his head a bit at this age. Allow him to grip your fingers and pull up slightly, just as the doctor does to test his strength. He will pull up slightly, but it is quite normal to still have some head lag while doing so. More active babies will have lots of movement, but it is too early to see real scooting or turning over.

My Regards

Your baby is now able to appreciate her environment in greater ways than before. She can make her needs known by the type of cry she makes. She will regard your face and the faces of others, and she will focus on many different objects. Your baby can now see and focus four to five feet away. Her vision is surely not 20/20 yet, but she can see you indeed! She will enjoy following all the members of her fan club as they pass!

I Love Mommy

Now is the time to see that wonderful social smile in response to your stimulation. He will respond to your voice and to the voices of others, in particular to those voices that he has heard frequently. Your baby will pay attention to different sounds and will follow them by turning his head toward them. He will love when you speak to him and engage him, so continue to do so daily and enjoy every sweet minute!

Feeding

How are you both doing with the feeding scene? By this time you should have settled into a fairly regular feeding routine. Hopefully your baby is awakening on her own during the day without needing you to wake her to feed. The night feedings may still be one, two, or three in number, especially if you are breast-feeding. On the other hand, at this age some babies are only up once per night after a late evening feeding. Continue to be boring and quiet with little stimulation during overnight feedings, and she will sleep for longer and longer intervals between feedings.

WHEN TO WEAN

If you are breast-feeding, how long is long enough? You may be wondering when to wean. There may be multiple factors you need to consider, such as a return to the workplace and your ongoing milk supply. Although many agencies (such as the World Health Organization and the American Academy of Pediatrics) may suggest weaning at four to six months, there are no hard-and-fast rules. This is a personal decision. When it is time to wean your baby, you will know, and the baby will be fine.

By now you should easily be able to discern your baby's cry for hunger. There is a quality to the cry that differs from others and that serves as a cue to feeding time. Remember that ritual and routine are invaluable for your baby now and in the future. Regular feedings are in place, and she has more wakeful time daily. Begin to think about a morning nap and an afternoon nap. She will need these breaks to rest during the day. Two-month-old babies require less sleep than newborns, but they still need quite a bit . . . much more than we do. Still, get your rest when you can—you must be healthy for your baby to be healthy!

DR. PETE'S ADVICE

NIGHT OWL

If your baby still has his days and nights confused get him on track by feeding him every three hours during the day, between 8 a.m. and 8 p.m. Awaken him by gently rubbing his cheeks or tickling his feet. Of course, feed sooner on demand if he awakens, but this is uncommon. Usually, you will have to awaken him to feed every three hours. Be certain to follow your normal routine. But . . . after 8 p.m., never wake a sleeping baby (unless you have been told that you need to for medical reasons) and only feed him on demand and do so in a dark, quiet place. Over time, he will think that his new family is wonderful, but so boring overnight that he will stretch the intervals between feedings with each passing week.

Personality Plus

You have now noticed more wakeful time after feedings. Your baby is more alert and aware of the world around him. Babies don't want to miss anything that is happening in their little world! Let them enjoy their environment. Two-month-old babies will not necessarily fall asleep at the close of each feeding as they did before. Try to put him down for naps and at bedtime while he is still somewhat awake.

Routines Rule

Make it a habit to cultivate the bedtime routine. You may want to think of a particular hour by which to accomplish the routine. For example, have the feeding, bath, book, song, and prayer all done and the baby in bed by eight o'clock.

Of course, personalize this routine, but by all means make it a routine that she can depend on. Regular, established ritual and routine will prevent later confusion and trauma for both you and your baby.

Keep it Up

Whether you have been breast-feeding or bottle-feeding with formula or expressed breast milk, you have been working hard. You should be very proud of yourself for the dedication this has taken for two months. You have clearly sustained her life with nutrition, and the gains in her measurements attest to that. Continue to interact as you feed your baby. She will thrive on nutrition given with large doses of your love.

Thriving Baby

Unless directed by your pediatrician, avoid adding anything to your baby's liquid diet at this age. A common old wives' tale suggests that adding cereal to a bottle will help the baby sleep better, but this can be counterproductive. Your baby is alert, growing, and thriving in all ways due to your loving care. Revel in that! Make time for yourself . . . remember that your baby will be happy and healthy if you are!

Hot Shots

It's time to vaccinate your baby now, and this time the recommendations call for several vaccines to be given. This protocol has been arrived at after years of ongoing research and refinement, and it is safe for your baby. Vaccines are again drawn up into syringes to be given intramuscularly. Be reassured that all of these vaccines are preservative-free, whether injectable or oral. The vaccines your baby receives are safe, and they directly stimulate his immune system. Vaccines give your baby antigens, in response to which he will make antibodies for his protection. His immune system will accept the antigen and begin to make the antibodies soon thereafter. Armed with antibodies, your baby will be protected when exposed to these infectious diseases.

At this visit she will receive another vaccination against hepatitis B. The second in the series, the dosage is the same. She should also receive a DTAP vaccine, which protects her from diphtheria, tetanus, and pertussis. These are all bacterial pathogens from which it is important to be protected, but pertussis, or whooping cough, can be life threatening if contracted in the first two years of life. The pneumococcal vaccine, or PCV, protects your baby from a dangerous, invasive streptococcal infection. She will also receive a vaccine against Hemophilus influenzae B. This is called the HIB vaccine. Despite the name, this serious bacterial pathogen is unrelated to influenza virus.

Next, your baby will receive the inactivated polio vaccine, or IPV. This will protect her from poliovirus,

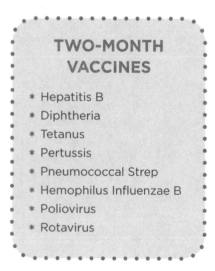

TWO-MONTH VACCINES

* Hepatitis B
* Diphtheria
* Tetanus
* Pertussis
* Pneumococcal Strep
* Hemophilus Influenzae B
* Poliovirus
* Rotavirus

which crippled many people, prior to the advent of the vaccine in the 1950s. Thankfully, vaccine protection has nearly eradicated this virus. Finally, she will receive one oral vaccine against rotavirus, a significant intestinal virus that can easily cause infants to get dehydrated and often requires admission to the hospital for intravenous fluids. Rest assured that the vaccines are safe for your baby and that you are protecting her from the evil of infectious diseases.

Thanks to much research and many clinical studies, many vaccines may be combined today. Combination vaccines are manufactured to contain more than one antigen. Some vaccines available today contain up to five in one. These vaccines are also preservative-free, and they are just as effective as the single-dose vaccines. The best news is that they allow your baby to have fewer injections. Less pain for your baby means fewer tears for both of you!

Once the vaccines have been administered, pick up your little guy and console him. He will calm with your soothing. Some moms wish to give a dose of pain reliever before or directly following the vaccinations, but this is not necessary. Reactions are mild, if present at all, and are confined to local swelling or tenderness, mild fussiness, and low-grade fever. If any reaction occurs, you may use warm compresses locally and the analgesic acetaminophen as needed for comfort.

What's Next?

As the two-month well baby visit comes to a close, your pediatrician will sit with you and summarize the checkup. During and after the full examination, the doctor will have pointed out to you any pertinent findings regarding your baby's body. She will explain the nature of these findings and let you know if there is anything to be concerned about. Be reassured that your feedings have successfully allowed your baby to grow and thrive, and her growth and developmental milestones attest to this, even after only two months of life.

DR. PETE'S ADVICE

TO SPIT OR NOT TO SPIT

Always report to your pediatrician if your baby is spitty, especially if it is a new occurrence. Spitty babies may have gastroesophageal reflux, which will resolve with time and a bit of help. Reflux is treated with elevation, thickened feeds, and medication (if indicated). Projectile vomiting exceeds spitting and may be an indication of pyloric stenosis. Seek evaluation right away.

Your feedings remain liquid, as it is not yet time to introduce solids into your baby's diet. Any exceptions to this will be discussed by your pediatrician. One common exception is gastroesophageal reflux, for which you may be advised to thicken any bottle-feedings. Projectile vomiting rarely occurs, but it must be reported immediately and followed up with an appointment at the doctor's office. Signs of teething are apparent, though the first teeth are usually seen after six months of age.

Your baby should have received his vaccinations, both injected and oral. Any necessary medications will be discussed, with the appropriate dosages given. It is best to write down this information if your doctor hasn't already done so. It is rare to need medication at this age. An analgesic may be used following the administration of vaccines, but only if the adverse effects warrant this for your baby's comfort. Use medication as a last resort . . . only if it is truly needed. Of course, we do want him to be comfortable. If you use acetaminophen, be certain to use the correct amount as advised by your pediatrician. If needed, acetaminophen can be administered every four hours.

Finally, before you leave, be certain that your concerns have been addressed and your questions answered.

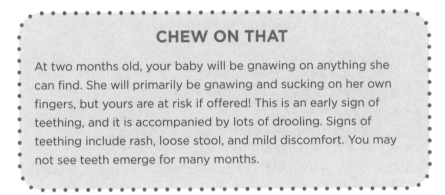

CHEW ON THAT

At two months old, your baby will be gnawing on anything she can find. She will primarily be gnawing and sucking on her own fingers, but yours are at risk if offered! This is an early sign of teething, and it is accompanied by lots of drooling. Signs of teething include rash, loose stool, and mild discomfort. You may not see teeth emerge for many months.

73

Final Questions

You have learned a lot at this visit, and you may have additional questions. Your doctor will surely address any of your concerns. She will show you the baby's growth chart, and if the growth curves are consistent, there are no concerns. Your baby's head size may still be out of proportion with his body.

You have now seen that your baby has grown and developed before your eyes. She is not only bigger in size, but her personality is also emerging, and she is aware of so much more taking place around her. Your pediatrician will review development and reassure you that your baby is age-appropriate in motor, speech, intellectual, and social areas. Again, if your doctor notes an area that is out of the normal range, she will address this with you. Conversely, if you are worried about any part of your baby's development, this is the time to ask the pediatrician about it. She may then tell you what developmental gains to look for in the upcoming two months prior to the next checkup. This will be the baby's homework, hopefully to be completed by four months of age.

QUESTIONS TO ASK

Now is the time to ask any questions that have not already been answered by the doctor:

* Is my baby's exam totally normal?
* Is she developmentally age-appropriate?
* Is she growing well?
* Does she need any medication?
* Are there any adverse effects to look for from the vaccine?
* When will she turn over?

Looking Ahead

Most four-month-olds will be even more social, and you will feel the connection between the two of you. She will have more to say, and she will chuckle or laugh at you and her siblings. She will move more and begin to try to roll over, but generally she won't succeed in this endeavor until six months of age. Enjoy these changes in development as you see them over the next two months!

CHAPTER SEVEN

Four-Month Wellness Visit

It's time to see the pediatrician for the four-month well-child visit. Your baby is growing and changing with each day. There is much to discuss! Once you are greeted and brought to the examination room, undress your baby down to the diaper and keep him warm until your doctor appears.

Your baby will be looking all about as she is now more alert and curious than ever. Once she is placed supine on the exam table, you may notice that she is uncomfortable, and she may begin to cry. Even at only four months old, babies can feel vulnerable when undressed and on the exam table. It is as if they recall the last visit, which culminated in multiple vaccinations!

Exam Time

After the nurse weighs and measures your baby, your pediatrician will once again proceed through a full examination. She will examine your four-month-old completely, including neurologically. Part of every examination is the evaluation of the nervous system, which is done in various ways. Your baby's normal neurologic function is manifested in his tone, his reflexes, and his strength. As your pediatrician pulls him up from the supine position, he should no longer have any head lag. Your doctor may check to see if your four-month-old is able to stand and bear his weight with support. Ignore the common old wives' tale that standing at this age promotes bowing of his legs; the opposite is true. Full extension of his legs will strengthen them over time and will actually help alleviate the bowing from his position in utero. He may be placed in a stationary walker with a tray for toys. He will enjoy flexing and extending his legs.

Your pediatrician will inspect the skin for new birthmarks, as some of these may emerge in the months following birth. Also, he may have a diaper rash, some atopic dermatitis, or eczema. The latter is often familial and is statistically more common in individuals with lighter, fairer coloration.

Your doctor will of course examine your baby's hair, fontanel, and scalp, and then the ears, eyes, nose, and throat. If the baby has congestion, she may ask you the duration. Chronic congestion may be a sign of an allergy or sensitivity to the milk protein in either breast milk or formula.

She will then listen to his chest, front and back, and gently palpate the abdomen. Some infants have an umbilical hernia, or an "outie," at

"RIDE 'EM COWBOY"

You will notice that your newborn baby has bowing of his lower legs. This is a tibial torsion that is quite normal as it is a result of the folded leg position that most babies have in the uterus. No treatment is necessary other than tincture of time. As your baby grows, bowing becomes less prominent by six to nine months of age. It is a myth that bearing weight after four months of age is harmful. Sitting in a stationary walker does not cause increased bowing. On the contrary, bearing weight strengthens the legs and leads to decreased bowing. As your baby becomes a toddler and bears weight the bowing of the lower legs self corrects, usually by the age of two years.

Bearing their weight does not worsen this; rather, it leads to resolution, even in Texas!

the cord site. This is usually self-limited and benign, with most resolving within two years when the muscles beneath the cord site tighten.

She will inspect genitalia and examine the extremities. Finally, the doctor will test the hips for dislocation with the Ortolani maneuver.

GET DOWN—GET FUNKY

You will be surprised by your baby's movements during the examination at this age. Some very active babies are trying to roll over, usually being stopped by an arm on the turning side. Your pediatrician is accustomed to moving targets at any age. It is expected. It is part of her specialty. The doctor will be assessing not only the body during the exam, but also the signs of development that your baby displays.

Growth and Development

Your baby's weight, length, and head circumference are most likely increasing. This will be reviewed at summary time as usual. Her developmental progress will be discussed, and hopefully she has done her homework. By four months of age, your baby has developed even more personality, and she should be a happy little gal most of the time, barring illness.

You may now notice gross motor functions as well as fine motor functions. She may be trying to roll over, achieving the halfway mark. Very few babies roll over at this age, but a few will, especially if they are active and smaller in size. She will stare at her hands and hold them together, and she may transfer an object from hand to hand, but this is done inadvertently

NOTEABLES

Date: _____

Age: _____

Weight: _____

Length: _____

Head Circumference: _____

Notes from Visit: _____

_____

_____

_____

_____

_____

_____

_____

_____

_____

at this age. Her grasp will be strong, and your baby will grab any object that is placed in her hand. She will reach for and bat at objects in front of her. She can now sit with support, and she will enjoy standing with your support, extending her legs and pushing with them.

Speech development can be divided into receptive (hearing and processing) and expressive (what she says). Your baby now hears and responds to sounds more readily than before. She should be easily engaged and responsive, with lots of babble, oohing, cooing, and laughter. She should make different sounds at different pitches.

Intellectually, she is well related to and more aware of her surroundings. Your pediatrician will be watching for her to appear well related as opposed to apathetic. The apathetic infant may be sullen, whereas the well-related infant will be happy. She will let you know when she is not content or feeling safe. At this age, you can more easily discern her needs and wants by her vocal tone and her cry.

Socially, your baby should be responsive to your voice and touch, and she should be happy and loving life with you!

|79

I AM CURIOUS

Your baby is very much aware of the world around her, including your home and all of her fans. You will be pleasantly surprised at her ability to focus on many different objects in her view. It's not too early to be reading books to stimulate her. You should do this at least once daily. Colorful toys and objects that she can reach for are good suggestions for further stimulation and enjoyment.

Feeding

During the first four months of your new baby's life, he has received a liquid diet. This has included breast milk or formula, or a combination of the two, and he has grown and thrived thanks to your care. So what comes next? Most experts agree that although it is not necessary to introduce solids at this age, the four-month-old infant's intestinal tract and digestive system are ready for solids and can handle them without event. One sign that your baby is ready for solids is obvious hunger in spite of more frequent breast- or bottle-feeding. Another sign of readiness for solids at four months is playfulness and prolonged feeding time with the breast or bottle, as they stop and go.

To begin, you may introduce two tablespoons of iron-fortified infant cereal twice daily. This is available as rice, oat, or barley cereal. Mix your

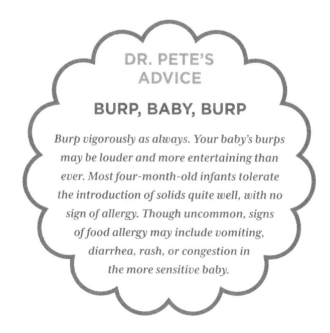

DR. PETE'S ADVICE

BURP, BABY, BURP

Burp vigorously as always. Your baby's burps may be louder and more entertaining than ever. Most four-month-old infants tolerate the introduction of solids quite well, with no sign of allergy. Though uncommon, signs of food allergy may include vomiting, diarrhea, rash, or congestion in the more sensitive baby.

expressed breast milk or formula with the cereal so that it has the consistency of oatmeal, which is handled better than loose and soupy cereal. Choose a morning and an evening feeding time that he is already accustomed to, and begin with the cereal, followed by breast- or bottle-feeding. Your baby will have the appetite and impetus to take the solid, and it will not detract from his usual feeding, although the time and volume of that feeding may decrease slightly.

As you introduce solids to your baby, be sure to take some fun pictures as he learns to feed in this new way. Your baby will be excited as you feed him, making funny faces as he learns to take in the solids. He may be impatient during the few seconds it takes to reload the spoon with his cereal or fruit. This is expected. Don't be anxious, and take your time. Most babies accept the smooth texture of stage-one solids with ease. Don't forget to involve your partner in the feeding scene. Both your baby and your partner will enjoy this!

It's best to use the same solid for three days, so that you may watch for signs of sensitivity. Allergic reactions are uncommon in general. There may be a higher incidence if there is a significant family history of food allergy. Introduce two tablespoons of stage-one infant fruits in the same manner, eventually giving cereal and fruit together twice daily. They may be given as alternative spoonfuls or even mixed on a spoonful.

Finally, beware of the potential change in stool pattern. Solids usually bring some expected changes in his diaper. Some solids are more binding, such as bananas, applesauce, and rice cereal. If your baby seems constipated after introducing solids, report this to your pediatrician.

Hot Shots

It's that time again. Your baby needs protection from illness, and vaccinations differ with each well visit. At four months of age, there is one less injection. The hepatitis B vaccine has been administered to your baby twice by now, and this vaccine will not be given again until she is nine months old.

At this visit, she should receive vaccination against diphtheria, tetanus, pertussis (DTAP), Hemophilus influenzae B (HIB), pneumococcal strep (PCV), poliovirus (IPV), and rotavirus. This means that your baby will receive four intramuscular injections and one oral vaccination. If your pediatrician is utilizing the combination vaccines, then she will only need to receive two injections. If this is the case, the DTAP, HIB, and IPV vaccinations may be combined in one syringe. This confers immunity just as effectively, and it is just as safe for your baby.

> ## FOUR-MONTH VACCINES
>
> The recommended vaccines at four months of age differ from those administered at the last well-baby visit. Here is the list:
>
> * Diphtheria
> * Tetanus
> * Pertussis
> * Pneumococcal strep
> * Hemophilus influenzae B
> * Rotavirus
> * Poliovirus

Most babies have no reactions to these vaccines, or the reaction is mild if present. Remember that mild reactions can include local swelling or tenderness and/or fussiness and low-grade temperature elevation. Babies register pain just as we do, and injections certainly yield discomfort. Their discomfort from each injection is brief, lasting as long as the needle is in, just a second or two. Once the vaccinations have been administered, pick her up to comfort and console her. Your comfort is all that she needs, and simply holding her, walking, and gently whispering is usually sufficient. If she needs more soothing, you may give her a feeding to help. Your doctor's office may have a separate room for this.

If your baby did not have any reaction after receiving her vaccines at two months of age, then the likelihood that she reacts adversely at this time is quite low. There is no guarantee, of course, so be prepared to apply warm compresses to her thigh as needed, and consider a dose of analgesic if she is fussy or warm to touch. You will already be dosing her with your tender loving care.

What's Next?

Now that your baby has been examined completely, your pediatrician will review the four-month well-baby visit with you. He will explain any new physical findings and review the baby's developmental progress. You will see her growth charts with the gains made in weight, length, and head circumference. The increases in each of these parameters should be affirming for you, as they are due to the excellent work that you have done in providing your baby with proper nutrition. Finally, your doctor will recommend any medication needed, render dietary advice, and let you know what developmental milestones to watch for next. It's time for reassurance and education, so hold on and enjoy!

Your doctor will review the exciting changes in diet with the introduction of solids. You have heard about cereal and fruit and those that can bind his stool, leading to discomfort from constipation. The most common culprits are rice cereal, bananas, and applesauce. Call the pediatric office for advice if constipation occurs.

Fruits purees can be prepared at home by those who have time and wish to do so. You may prepare these in your kitchen, using fruits such as apples, bananas, pears, and peaches. The fruits should be blanched, peeled, and food-processed with water or breast milk or formula so as to achieve a smooth, pureed texture. These homemade solids can be stored in the freezer in ice-cube trays for easy pop-out helpings. Your baby will still burp, but there is no need to spend a long time seeking that burp.

Food allergy is uncommon, but you need to be aware of the signs and symptoms.

Dads need and want to help, so avail yourself of their help, and let the big brother and/or big sister help with your baby's care as well. Dads and siblings will love to help with the feedings! When dads or partners are available and are allowed to help with your baby's care, you are both given a gift. The partner's gift is bonding and feeling needed by both of you, and your gift is the respite from your constant care-giving.

At this age your baby will enjoy being upright, but the use of walkers is controversial. Infants who use walkers do not walk any sooner. Nor do walkers delay walking, as long as the baby is not spending too much time in it. Injuries and even deaths have prompted pediatricians to discourage the use of mobile walkers. Please use a stationary walker or a jumper. These are fun and entertaining for your baby without placing him at risk. Mobile walkers find stairs to travel down!

JUICING

Pediatricians are often asked if there is a specific time to introduce fruit juice into an infant's diet. Juice is actually not necessary to your baby's diet. Juice provides empty calories. Juice is sweet. Introducing juice too early may also reduce your baby's desire to take her milk regularly. However, your doctor may advise you to provide diluted juice if your baby is suffering from constipation.

Final Questions

There may be more issues to discuss before your visit is complete. Developmentally, your curious little one is watching every move you make and is enjoying and responding to all kinds of sounds. How thrilling for you to hear that she is age-appropriate in her motor skills and speech development.

At this age, you have seen her more alert, aware, seeing farther away, and following more actively. She is trying to roll over, and may have already done so in one direction. She may be trying to push herself up when in the prone position. Your baby now enjoys being pulled up and standing with your support, and she has good head and neck tone.

Socially, she is showing more personality, and you should feel a special connection with your little one. Lots of chuckling happens in response to all of her fans! She should be bonding not only with you, but also with her daddy or your partner as they interact as well.

Vaccines have been given, or they may follow this review, and they should have been explained thoroughly, along with any potential reactions that you may see in your baby.

Your pediatrician may discuss common skin conditions such as eczema, also known as atopic dermatitis, especially if it has appeared. Eczema is a common skin condition that can affect infants, children, and adults. It is inflammatory in nature. Eczema is quite often a familial trait, with a history of eczema on one or both sides of the family. Patches that are pink or red and dry or scaly can affect the skin on any part of the body. The hallmark of therapy is to moisturize. Your pediatrician may prescribe anti-inflammatory medication for persistent problem areas.

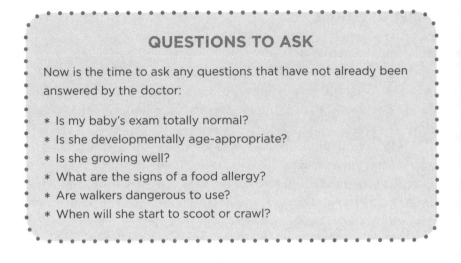

QUESTIONS TO ASK

Now is the time to ask any questions that have not already been answered by the doctor:

* Is my baby's exam totally normal?
* Is she developmentally age-appropriate?
* Is she growing well?
* What are the signs of a food allergy?
* Are walkers dangerous to use?
* When will she start to scoot or crawl?

86

Looking Ahead

Watch for many new signs of normal development by six months of age. At six months, your baby may be purposely transferring an object from hand to hand, performing press-ups with her head held high when prone, and reaching for objects and actually grabbing them! Listen for sing-song screeching and even more laughing. She should be well related and more aware. She may be a social butterfly, or she may begin to show signs of stranger anxiety. Finally, make certain that your questions are answered, and if you have forgotten any, simply call the office at any time.

CHAPTER EIGHT

Six-Month Wellness Visit

How time flies! Your baby is now six months old and halfway to her first birthday! You have come so far, and you should be very proud of yourself. You have learned a great deal, and you have cared for her lovingly. By now you are probably more relaxed and at ease.

When you enter your pediatrician's office, you will again be greeted by the staff, who will know you and your baby, especially if you have been in the office for other issues. She will be weighed and measured, and she will then be examined by her doctor. Expect that she will be more active than ever, and it is a toss-up how she will react to the office staff and to her pediatrician. She may be quite social, but your baby may also shriek! Many babies begin a phase of development known as stranger anxiety, during which they are fearful of strangers, so don't be alarmed or surprised. This is quite normal.

Exam Time

When your pediatrician examines your baby, he will begin with the head, neck, hair, and scalp. Hair growth may prevent the easy inspection of the past. Your doctor will look for any new lesions on the skin. Some "birthmarks" will appear in these months following birth. The doctor will listen to her chest for heart sounds and lung sounds. He will palpate your baby's abdomen to check for any organ enlargement, and he will inspect the genitalia for normal growth. The arms and legs will be tested for reflexes and strength. This might not be easy, because your little gal may be actively trying to roll over during the examination! The doctor will stand her up to see how she bears weight with support and to look at her back. He may do a horizontal lift to evaluate her tone. Your baby should hold up her head and her pelvis while held in this position.

Do I Measure Up?

It is once again time for your baby to be measured. This includes her length, her weight, and her head circumference. The head circumference is actually the most important measurement of the three, denoting the ongoing growth of the brain. Don't be surprised if she is a moving target, as she may have mastered the rollover maneuver by this age. You will want to see consistent growth velocity in all areas . . . don't concentrate on the percentiles.

What Is Auscultation?

Auscultation may be a large word, but it simply means the act of listening to sounds in the body. Your pediatrician can auscultate, or listen to sounds in the chest and the abdomen, with the stethoscope. He may rub the head of the stethoscope in his hand. Friction will warm it before he places it on your baby's skin. He will auscultate the chest for heart sounds and lung sounds. He may auscultate the abdomen to listen for normal bowel sounds.

What Is Palpation?

Palpation is the act of feeling with the hand. The doctor palpates by applying light pressure with his fingers on the surface of the body. This allows him to determine the consistency of the parts beneath the surface. The doctor will palpate your baby's lymph nodes or glands throughout the body. He will also palpate the neck to evaluate the thyroid gland. Abdominal palpation is routine, evaluating the liver, spleen, and intestinal tract, and monitoring for the rare finding of a mass (a growth, such as a cyst or tumor).

NOTEABLES

Date: _____

Age: _____

Weight: _____

Length: _____

Head Circumference: _____

Notes from Visit: _____

_____

_____

_____

_____

_____

_____

_____

_____

_____

DR. PETE'S ADVICE

"BIGGER ISN'T BETTER"

When reviewing growth, pediatricians always stress the importance of consistent growth velocity, and being reasonably well proportioned. Every infant or child is unique and special. Healthy physical growth for each one is to grow along his own growth curve for height, weight, and head circumference. Family history of size and stature weighs in heavily on this (no pun intended!). So please don't think that the child who is in the 95th percentile for his growth parameters will be any more successful in life than the one who is in the 5th percentile.

Put away the Yale tee shirts and concentrate upon consistent growth along their own growth curve, no matter where it is on the chart.

Growth and Development

Your baby has been weighed, measured, and fully examined at this visit, and now you will be shown his growth charts. He should have good, consistent growth velocity since the last visit. In terms of developmental progress, it is wonderful to see your little one becoming even more responsive to you and interactive with you each day!

Motorically, he may be rolling over one or both ways by now, and he should not have any head lag as you pull him to the sitting position by his hands. Your six-month-old should be using his arms to prop himself up when he is in the prone position. Press-ups are accomplished first, with arms pressing up and supporting the chest, and with the waist and legs remaining down. The press-up position leads to rolling over, usually from front to back first. Over the next one to three months, he will probably roll over from front to back, and then from back to front. He may even begin to scoot backward while supine. He will begin to get much more mobile! He probably loves to find and play with his toes! Transferring objects from hand to hand with purpose begins now, and he can reach with accuracy. Your baby will enjoy standing if you hold him up and he can sit with a bit of support.

With regard to speech and language development, he should be very vocal, with frequent sing-song high-pitched sounds, in addition to the babble that you have come to love. You will notice that he will speak more often and for longer periods of time.

Intellectually, your six-month-old will show signs of understanding concepts. He may hold and study one toy with great concentration, or he may notice that a toy is behind another and try to reach it. He may also show displeasure at the loss of a toy. He may or may not respond to the calling of his name. Not to worry.

Socially, your baby should be increasingly responsive with you and with others, unless stranger anxiety has set in. Stranger anxiety is common and is usually restricted to those he sees infrequently. It may last one to three months. It is normal. This too shall pass. He will now show a variety of emotions, and he can easily react to your emotions as well, whatever they may be. He should be a happy little guy most of the time, as long as he is receiving proper nutrition and rest. Six-month-olds can exhibit many moods and emotions, just as we do, including shyness, happiness, fear, and disappointment.

He may enjoy seeing his reflection in a mirror, and he can now self-soothe.

Purposeful Play

What fun to have toys to have and to hold. Be certain that they are safe and age-appropriate. Your baby will enjoy concentrating on individual toys, and he may seem to have a favorite or two. At this age, he should transfer a toy from hand to hand with purpose. Prior to this point, a transfer was likely to be inadvertent. If a toy is just out of reach, it may prompt him to reach and scoot toward the toy. He will become more mobile each day!

TEETHING TIPS

Your baby is now actively teething, and this can be uncomfortable. You may use an analgesic if needed. He will enjoy gnawing on cool teething rings or on half of a hard, stale bagel. Avoid the use of topical numbing agents; if overused, they may temporarily affect his swallowing function. Teething may be associated with rash, loosened stool, and intermittent bouts of fussiness from discomfort.

Feeding

At six months of age, your baby is probably enjoying her solid foods two or three times daily. She may be devouring cereal and fruit, and hopefully she is tolerating it quite well. It is fun to see babies enjoy solids and learn to receive them from a spoon. Most six-month-old babies acclimate to spoon-feeding without difficulty. If you feel that she is hesitant to feed in this way, or if you feel that she has any discomfort with swallowing, please report this to your pediatrician. Some babies will take more time to master spoon-feeding, and that is normal.

If your baby is not already consuming vegetables, she can receive them at this age. Stage-one vegetables may be found at the store, and they will have the texture of a puree. Of course, you can prepare you own vegetables for her if you wish. In the spirit of giving two solids at a sitting, serve the vegetables with yogurt or pastina. If you are currently giving her solids in the morning and evening, she can have her vegetables midday. Yogurt should be smooth and custard-style, with no chunks of fruit, which may cause choking. You can prepare the pastina with a hint of butter.

At six months old, your baby may begin receiving meats for the first time! This is best in the evening (dinnertime), and it may replace the evening cereal. Your baby no longer needs cereal twice daily. You can prepare meats at home; they are also available commercially with the other infant foods.

93

It is not too early to think of a five-feeding schedule with an early milk feeding, three solid meals, and a late milk feeding, either from the breast or bottle. A schedule at this age will provide structure and a reliable pattern for you and your baby going forward.

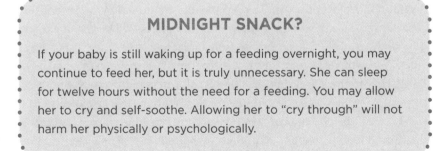

MIDNIGHT SNACK?

If your baby is still waking up for a feeding overnight, you may continue to feed her, but it is truly unnecessary. She can sleep for twelve hours without the need for a feeding. You may allow her to cry and self-soothe. Allowing her to "cry through" will not harm her physically or psychologically.

Open Wide

By now your baby loves to open wide for her solid foods. Remember to follow up the solids with breast milk or formula until she takes enough solids to be content. Solids do contain water. When she takes a solid meal without a chaser of milk, she will still be well hydrated. Remember that her stool will change depending on the solids she has taken in. This is normal.

Cereal, fruits, and vegetables are all well tolerated by most six-month-old babies. You can reduce her cereal to one serving each day. You can give her fruit twice daily as before. You can give her vegetables midday or in the evening, along with yogurt or pastina. Smooth, custard-style yogurt is best. Pastina may be found in the pasta section at the grocery store.

You can introduce meat to your baby at this age, usually at dinnertime, when you are dining as well! You may prepare basic meats in your kitchen by adding water or milk and using a food processor or blender. There is no real magic to the order of solids as long as she is receiving cereal, fruit, vegetables, and meat daily.

Choose your pattern and stick to it in order to lessen confusion and maintain consistency.

Hot Shots

It's time for protection again! The vaccine recommendations at six months of age differ slightly, so let us review them. Your baby will receive the third dose of the diphtheria vaccine, as well as the tetanus and pertussis vaccines. You will recall that these are combined, and they are known as DTAP. The letter A stands for "acellular." This refers to the way the pertussis portion of the vaccine is manufactured. Your baby will also receive the third dose of the pneumococcal strep vaccine. In addition, he will receive the third dose of Hemophilus influenzae B protection. The latter two are single-dose vaccines. An exception occurs if your pediatrician is utilizing combination vaccines. Finally, he will also receive the third and final dose of rotavirus vaccine, the one administered orally.

The five-in-one vaccine contains diphtheria, tetanus, pertussis, poliovirus, and Hemophilus. If this is given, rest assured that the combination vaccine is preservative-free, safe, and equally effective to confer immunity to your baby. If the five-in-one vaccine is used, your baby will only receive two injections, again in the anterior part of his thigh. However, if the combination vaccine is not used, he will receive three injections: DTAP, HIB, and pneumococcal strep. You will notice that when the combination vaccine is used, poliovirus is included in the dose. When the combination vaccine is not used, your baby does not need to receive a third dose of poliovirus (IPV). The dose is optional at this age.

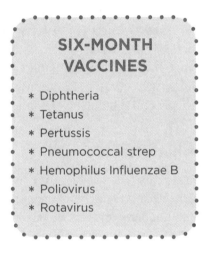

SIX-MONTH VACCINES

* Diphtheria
* Tetanus
* Pertussis
* Pneumococcal strep
* Hemophilus Influenzae B
* Poliovirus
* Rotavirus

Is there such a thing as too much vaccine? In general, too little vaccine is ill advised because you wish for your baby to have full immunity to infectious diseases. In the case of four versus five polio vaccines to complete a series, it is not bad to have more . . . it simply means that more antibodies are created. In fact, in the case of questionable vaccine status in babies adopted from foreign countries, vaccines are commonly repeated. More vaccine has not been shown to cause any harm.

No Pain, No Gain

Once again, your baby will receive injections directly into his muscle. The anterior part of the thigh is used again, as it was at four months of age. The injection is given at a slight angle so as not to reach the femur (bone).

Intramuscular injections are rapidly absorbed. They are painful, but the discomfort is short-lived.

At this age, your baby is more aware of his surroundings than ever. Consolation in your arms is even more meaningful now because he is acutely aware of what has occurred. One day he will realize all that you did to protect him from illness and life-threatening infections. Relish your role of protector, his main advocate for his ongoing health and wellness.

Once the injections have been given to your baby, he may be dressed for departure. The injection sites may display a drop of blood, or they may not. Either is acceptable. If there is a drop of blood at the site, the nurse or doctor will clean the site. Applying a Band-Aid to the oozing injection site will prevent spots on his clothing.

What's Next?

Your pediatrician will now review the six-month well-baby visit with you. Some doctors do this after the injections have been administered, but most will summarize the visit and leave the injections for the last minute. By this time, he will have reviewed your baby's growth, looking for a gal who is well-proportioned with consistent growth over time. This wonderful growth is due to the nutrition you alone have provided, and that is about to change! Your baby is probably enjoying solids now, and it's time to add a few things to the menu. Cereal and fruit may be given in the morning, vegetables with yogurt or pastina may be given midday, and now meat, vegetables, and fruit may be given at dinnertime. She will still require the first morning feeding of breast milk or formula, as well as the last evening feeding of the same.

You have learned that she no longer needs to feed through the night, and hopefully everyone in the family is sleeping through the night. It is wise to settle into such a pattern for consistency. Your baby will anticipate feeding times, and daily life will have a sense of order that you both may rely on.

Where are those teeth? Your baby has been drooling and gnawing for months, and perhaps there are still no teeth in sight. This is normal. First teeth may be seen between three and sixteen months, on the average appearing at six or seven months of age. The two lower central incisors are usually the first to be seen, followed by the upper central incisors. There is no medical significance to this timing . . . some babies teethe early and some teethe late.

Yogurt
You may give your baby yogurt if you wish. The yogurt should be smooth and custard-style. Avoid yogurt with pieces of fruit, as this could cause your baby to choke. You may use plain or flavored yogurts. Fruit-flavored yogurt is processed and rarely causes reactions. The yogurt that you choose need not be specialized for infants. He may take low-fat yogurt that you eat. Watch the labels, as some brands of yogurt are too high in sugar content.

Pastina
Pastina is egg pasta in tiny star shapes and can be found at the grocery store. It is prepared like any other pasta, with a small amount of melted butter mixed into it. Pastina may be given separately or in combination with the vegetable on the spoon. The texture will be new to your baby; he may reject it initially . . . it may be drying on your wallpaper!

Meat Lovers
Meats can be introduced at this age and are generally well tolerated. Single meats are available at the grocery store, and all are FDA-approved. They are available in many varieties, and they vary in their palatability. Unless you prepare your own, try the jars of meat and vegetable combinations for better taste.

Final Questions

You have learned and seen much with regard to your baby's development, and she has become more social, alive, and aware with each day. As long as your pediatrician reassures you that your baby is in the normal range for all of her developmental milestones, all is well. Every baby is different, and they all have different personalities. Don't be surprised that siblings usually differ greatly as well. Your baby may or may not have begun to show signs of stranger anxiety, but if so, this is quite normal and usually passes within several months. There is no treatment for this normal stage in her development. Reassure those with whom she is anxious . . . they should not take it personally! This too shall pass.

QUESTIONS TO ASK

Now is the time to ask any questions that have not already been answered by the doctor:

* Is my baby's exam totally normal?
* Is she developmentally age-appropriate?
* Is she growing well?
* When will my baby crawl?
* When will we see her teeth come in?

She has become more alert, curious, and active than ever, and you have seen that she transfers objects with ease and purpose, she has probably begun to roll over, and she loves finding and playing with her toes. The toes may be drawn up to her mouth for a tasting! She is now more mobile than ever, and she will be trying to scoot to move from place to place. This usually occurs on the back first. Smaller, thinner babies have an easier time with this activity, but this does not mean that they are more advanced. Your baby is now more vocal; she has a lot to say, and she wants to be heard, so everyone should listen up!

Looking Ahead

Watch for many new signs of development by nine months of age. Your baby will change greatly in the next three months. Watch for scooting to become crawling, although some babies skip the crawling stage and simply pull up to the standing position. This is normal. She will become more vocal, and by the next visit she should be forming monosyllables, or one-syllable utterances. These should not be in context, and they will be repeated, as they enjoy hearing themselves! For example, "la, la, la, ba, ba, ba, da, da, da," etc.

THE STRAWBERRY

This common birthmark, bright and beautiful and red, is called a hemangioma. It is benign. A hemangioma is vascular, meaning that it is comprised of growing blood vessels. They are painless. Capillary hemangiomas are above the skin, and cavernous hemangiomas are below the skin. Hemangiomas increase in size until about nine months of age, and then they have slow, steady resolution.

Creepy Crawly

Infants usually learn to crawl between six and nine months of age, but some may not. Scooting is the first step on the way to crawling; this starts when they are supine, or on their back. When prone, or tummy down, he will begin to army crawl, followed by the four-point crawl. Some babies skip crawling altogether and pull up to their knees, and then pull to the standing position.

Chit Chat

Your baby is probably vocalizing actively at six months of age. A variety of sounds can be heard. In addition to crying, she will be laughing, screeching, squealing, babbling, and constantly responding to your voice. You will notice that she uses different sounds for the various emotions she is displaying.

Over the next three months, you should notice development of single-syllable utterances, though not in context as yet.

CHAPTER NINE

Nine-Month Wellness Visit

Unless your baby needed evaluation for an illness, three months have passed since the last well-baby visit at your pediatrician's office. He has grown and thrived because of your care. You will enter the office as always, the staff will greet you, and someone will take you to an examination room. A nurse will weigh and measure your baby before the examination begins.

At this age, your baby may be insecure and fearful if left sitting alone on a scale or exam table. Your pediatrician may choose to have you hold your baby on your lap. This allows him to be with you and to take comfort in your touch, your smell, and your reassuring words. He will feel more safe and secure and less vulnerable on your lap. Your doctor will guide you as to the proper way to hold your baby as the exam progresses. It's also prudent to keep him secure, as this is the time that separation anxiety may begin.

Exam Time

As always, the examination begins at the top of the head and extends down to the toes. The anterior fontanel should be smaller and thicker as it fibroses, and your pediatrician will inspect his hair and scalp. She will also inspect the face, eyes, ears, nose, mouth, and throat, and she will probably see some new teeth! She will examine his neck and listen to his chest for normal breath sounds and heart sounds. Your pediatrician will palpate the abdomen as well, seeking normal-sized organs with no tenderness. Again, she will examine the genitalia. She will then test the arms and legs for strength and elicit normal reflexes. Finally, the doctor will evaluate your baby's general tone.

How Do You Do?

Your baby is very social and interactive now, but he may not want you to let him go. Separation anxiety is common, and it may begin at nine months of age. This anxiety can occur when you are not holding him or if you are not in his sight. Reassure your partner and other family members that this will pass in a few months; no one should take this personally. This phase of development is quite normal and often follows the phase of stranger anxiety. For one to three months, he may want only you. This too shall pass. . . .

On the Lap

The most secure position for your baby is right on your lap. This is a suitable place to have his examination. Your pediatrician will sit close to your baby and interact with him as she examines him. Different positions will be achieved easily, as your lap functions as the examination table. He will be most comfortable and secure with you; therefore, he will be more at ease and quieter for a more accurate exam by your doctor.

The successful exam of an active and perhaps fearful nine-month-old depends on the holder. Your pediatrician will guide you as to the most appropriate holding position for the part of the body that is being examined. For example, turning your baby to the side-saddle position, held close to your chest, allows for a pain-free evaluation of each ear. A reclined forward-facing position on your lap will allow an accurate examination of his abdomen.

Keep On Ticking

The examination of your baby's heart sounds is a fine art, as it is best done when he is quiet. Even though he is on your lap, he may still cry and be fearful. This is normal. Your pediatrician may try distraction techniques

NOTEABLES

Date: _____

Age: _____

Weight: _____

Length: _____

Head Circumference: _____

Notes from Visit: _____

_____

_____

_____

_____

_____

_____

_____

_____

_____

to try to calm and soothe your baby if he is upset. She has been trained to fully and thoroughly examine moving targets and loud patients. Not to worry.

Growth and Development

Your nine-month-old is on the go, full of life, and bringing you great joy each day. Your baby's motor development should be progressing steadily to include the scoot, creep, and crawl. Most have pulled to stand, and your baby may be cruising, which is sidestepping while holding onto something such as a coffee table or sofa—or your leg! It is usually too early to see them let go and balance. Your baby will likely enjoy taking steps while you are holding both of her hands in support. At this age, most babies can get to the sitting position on their own, and they are able to sit without support. The tripod sitting position is one in which her legs are apart with her arms on the floor in between as a prop. Your nine-month-old should be able to move about the room with a combination of roll and crawl maneuvers. She can now reach and find toys, even if they are hidden. She will enjoy throwing or dropping toys in repetition.

Your baby's speech development should include many monosyllables, with "da" being one of the easiest—and therefore the earliest—for you to hear from her. We allow dads to think this is directed toward them, although it is usually not in context as yet! She will love to repeat the da, ba, la, ga, and ma sounds.

Socially, your baby may begin to wave and clap her hands, especially if she sees you doing it often. Many respond to their name at this age and will wish to explore, touching anything, including your eyes, nose, and mouth! Intellectually, you will delight in seeing that she is still well related to her loved ones and to her surroundings. For example, she will look upward when she hears a plane, or she will look for dad when she hears the front door open at night.

Separation anxiety is common, and it can be seen between nine and fifteen months of age. She may be fearful when you leave her touch or her sight. The cause for this is a normal developmental milestone called object permanence. This is her realization that something exists even when it can't be seen (in this case, you). She realizes that you are not with her when she cannot see you. She wants you back! Proceed with your usual routine. She will not be harmed if she cries when you must go to the bathroom! This too shall pass.

DANGER, DANGER

Your baby's increased mobility can lead to increased risk for injury in and out of your home. The crawling and cruising infant can easily find stairs and sharp edges in the home as she wanders and explores. She may also be attracted to water outside, such as in a pool or the ocean. This is an appropriate time to revisit all the childproofing that was done prior to her birth. Inside your home, consider additional childproofing measures such as applying temporary rubber edges to cover a fireplace hearth. Outside your home, be extra vigilant.

Feeding

At this age, your baby wants nothing more than to eat your food. Some babies even go on a hunger strike with baby food until you reward them with your table food. Well, he is in luck, because you may now give table food to your baby. You need to be aware of certain guidelines before you begin. First, the fingers are the utensils of choice, but you should also allow him to practice holding a spoon. Table foods are acceptable as long

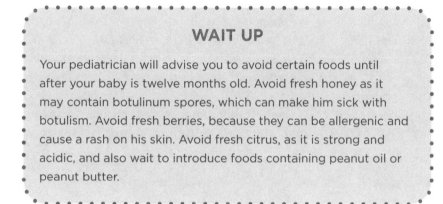

WAIT UP

Your pediatrician will advise you to avoid certain foods until after your baby is twelve months old. Avoid fresh honey as it may contain botulinum spores, which can make him sick with botulism. Avoid fresh berries, because they can be allergenic and cause a rash on his skin. Avoid fresh citrus, as it is strong and acidic, and also wait to introduce foods containing peanut oil or peanut butter.

as they are mashed or minced pieces. Be careful not to allow him any food large enough to lodge and cause a choking episode.

You may give him food as you have prepared it for the family; no need to make his plain or unseasoned. At this age, he will probably enjoy a variety of food textures. If you observe a particular aversion, report it to your pediatric office.

As he finger-feeds, you will notice the development of his pincer grasp. This is evident as he picks up individual oat rings to eat them. There are only a few foods to avoid, as discussed in the "Wait Up" advice above. Please purchase diphenhydramine, an antihistamine suspension, to have at home in case there is an allergic reaction to a newly ingested food. If an allergic reaction occurs, be certain to tell your pediatrician, and of course avoid offering this food again.

A multivitamin will be recommended to supplement vitamins A, D, C, and B complex, with fluoride for his dental enamel (unless fluoride is provided in your town's water). Most pediatricians advise breast milk or formula until twelve months of age, but yours may suggest whole milk at nine months. Most infants tolerate whole milk well, and combined with table food and a multivitamin, they have a balanced diet.

It is now time to introduce cups. Pediatric dentists favor straw-type sip cups to ensure proper facial muscular and palatal development. And given enough time, he should practice with your open cup for sips of milk or water. Be certain not to let go . . . he will pour it out with ease! Breast milk, formula, juice, water, or whole milk may be given by cup as opposed to the bottle. Give yourself a goal of six months to transition from bottles to full cup usage.

Hot Shots

At nine months old, your baby is active, mobile, and strong. Hold her firmly when she receives the vaccine. The vaccine at this visit may be given in the deltoid, or shoulder muscle, on either side. Your pediatrician may choose this muscle over the usual thigh site because there will be less discomfort later. There will be less discomfort because your baby is using her shoulder muscles much less than the thigh muscles now. She is probably pulling to stand, or standing when placed on her feet, and this means using those thigh muscles . . . we don't want them to be sore from the vaccine!

NINE-MONTH VACCINES

The recommended vaccines at nine months of age differ from those given at the last well-baby visit. Here is the list:

* Hepatitis B

Yes, that is correct. Your baby's immunization status is up-to-date. He only needs one vaccine at this visit, and that is the third and final hepatitis B vaccine. This vaccine is safe and carries no risk of significant adverse effects.

Vitamins

As you know, your breast-fed baby was supplemented with vitamins A, D, and C. Your formula-fed baby did not require this. All nine-month-old babies should have a supplement of vitamins A, D, C, and now vitamin B complex. This supplemental multivitamin is given via a one-milliliter dropper to the mouth and will help to provide her with a balanced dietary intake. Some babies love the taste of the multivitamin, and some do not. It is strong-smelling, but not at all harmful to her.

Your pediatrician will recommend a fluoride supplement for your baby to receive on a daily basis. This is most important to prevent dental caries (cavities), especially in the first ten years of life when tooth enamel is developing.

When prescribed in recommended doses, fluoride is safe for your baby, and it may be combined with the multivitamin. She should not receive fluoride simultaneously with milk, as the fluoride will not be as effective for her. Administer the fluoride, or vitamin with fluoride, either an hour before or an hour after any dairy intake.

What's Next?

It is again time to review and summarize this well-baby visit with your pediatrician. She will review your baby's growth and his physical examination, which hopefully was without any significant findings. If there are any abnormal findings on his examination, she will fully explain the concern and make any recommendations needed.

You have learned much about the allowable dietary changes at this age, and he will be so happy to be sharing your food. By now he should be sleeping through the night. If not, you should let him cry himself to sleep. He will learn to self-soothe, unless he is ill or in discomfort from active teething.

Table food is fundamental, and he will learn to self-feed with time. Begin to introduce drinking from a cup, first with a sip cup and then with an open cup—don't let go of the latter! Call your local community hospital or ambulance corps to inquire about available courses in infant resuscitation. Seek a class on infant choking, during which you and your partner may learn the infant Heimlich maneuver. You will then be prepared for the occasional choking episode, or the rare case of a lodged food particle. You will be more confident and you will remain calm if this ever occurs.

BE PREPARED

You will now be giving table food, and although it will be mashed or minced, your baby may gag and have a choking episode. If this occurs, you must be prepared. Do not panic. Pick him up and make certain that he is breathing. Hold him facedown in your arms, allowing gravity and his own efforts to compensate. Gently pat his back for reassurance. If an item is lodged, you may need to perform the infant Heimlich maneuver.

I Want to Talk

Your baby is ever so social, and he has a great deal to tell you. He wants to be heard! At this age the language is jargon or babble, only understood fully by your baby. He should be forming monosyllables and repeating them, though not in context as yet. Watch for more babble, laughter, and possibly one word in context by twelve months (hopefully it's "mama")!

I Want to Walk

Gross motor development can take off quickly for some nine- to twelve-month-olds. By now you have probably seen him crawl quickly, pull to stand, and cruise. If not, it should happen soon. Allow him the freedom to explore, ensuring that he always has a safe environment in which to move. Walk with him while holding his hands as he steps. Do not pull him up by the hands or wrists, as this can cause injury such as a radial head dislocation or "nursemaid's elbow." Hyperextension of an arm can result in the head of the radius (one of the bones in the forearm) being pulled out of the pocket of muscle in which it is seated. The arm hangs limp until a relocation of the bone is performed by your pediatrician.

I Want My Peers

Thus far your baby has interacted with you and the other adults in his life. Perhaps he has siblings or he is in a day care center, both of which are ideal for socialization. If not, please consider exposing your baby to those his age, so that he may socialize with peers. Don't worry about sharing germs; for his ongoing social development, the benefits outweigh the risks.

CAFÉ AU LAIT

The café au lait spot that you may see on your baby's skin is a benign birthmark. The name is French for "coffee with milk," because that is the color of this birthmark. It is a flat, harmless, painless, tan-colored spot that may appear at birth or during childhood in various shapes and sizes. Three or four of these are common in normal children. Six or more of these spots may be a sign of an inherited disorder called neurofibromatosis.

Final Questions

At this visit your pediatrician once again assessed your baby's developmental progress in the areas of gross motor skills, fine motor skills, receptive speech, expressive speech, and intellectual and social development. If your baby is anything but age-appropriate, your doctor will address the matter and fully explain the concern.

He may wish to observe your baby over time, or he may provide a referral for an evaluation. Please remember that you should try not to compare with friends or relatives. Every baby develops at his or her own rate, and there is a wide range of what is considered normal. Your pediatrician will tell you if you need to worry—never waste worry!

Your baby is probably cruising by now. If so, remember to ensure her safety inside and outside your home. Make certain that you readjust her car seat so that the restraints fit properly as she grows.

She is probably very social, but remember that separation anxiety is normal at this age, and you may desensitize her by allowing her to cry as you carry about your normal routine. She will not be harmed physically or emotionally. She will never doubt your love. She will not feel forgotten or forsaken.

Enjoy shopping for her first toothbrush, and make tooth-brushing a twice-daily part of her routine. Establishing the habit at this age will ensure fewer or no battles with a two-year-old!

Let Me Brush

As soon as your baby has teeth, it is time to purchase her very own toothbrush. You should make brushing teeth a part of her routine twice a day, and it should be a routine she will look forward to. Although there are infant toothpastes on the market, it is not necessary to use anything other than water. After she has brushed (played) by herself, you must then brush for her for a few seconds. Then you are done!

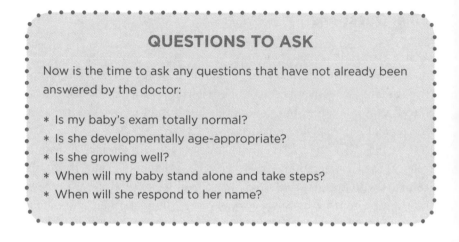

QUESTIONS TO ASK

Now is the time to ask any questions that have not already been answered by the doctor:

* Is my baby's exam totally normal?
* Is she developmentally age-appropriate?
* Is she growing well?
* When will my baby stand alone and take steps?
* When will she respond to her name?

Looking Ahead

Watch for many new signs of development by twelve months of age. These may include letting go to stand alone and balance, and becoming adept with real eating utensils. He may wave "bye-bye" and play "peek-a-boo" or "so big." He will become more active, and he will show even more of his unique personality.

CHAPTER TEN

Twelve-Month Wellness Visit

Congratulations! Happy first birthday to all of you! You have both made it! It has been twelve months since your baby's birth, and all is well. It's time once again to see your pediatrician for examination, evaluation, education, and affirmation. You have gone to great lengths as a new (or not-so-new) mother, and you should be very proud of all that you accomplished in the past year.

Once you have been greeted and seated at the office, your baby will be weighed and measured as always. Her head circumference is measured after her length and weight have been measured.

Exam Time

Your pediatrician will probably wish to examine your baby on your lap, as he did at the last examination at nine months of age. You will recall that this is wise in order to keep her as calm as possible for an accurate exam. She may be fearful with her doctor, and this is quite normal. On the other hand, some one-year-olds are not fearful, and they may enjoy the entire experience with laughter, interacting with the pediatrician from the beginning.

As usual, the doctor will examine from stem to stern . . . the head comes first, beginning with an inspection of her hair and scalp. He will survey the entire integument (skin) for any signs of inflammation, such as eczema, and for any new birthmarks that may have appeared. He will assess any new changes in birthmarks already known to be present. Your doctor will then examine her face, eyes, ears, nose, mouth, and throat thoroughly. He will test the neck for a normal range of motion and perform neck palpation for glands (lymph nodes). He will again listen to the chest to confirm normal heart and lung sounds. He will examine your baby's abdomen, or palpate in all four quadrants to make certain there is no organ enlargement. Finally, he will examine all four extremities (arms and legs) for strength, tone, and reflexes.

Remember to jot down any questions or concerns so that you will not forget them. Your baby will be active and keep you busy this time!

Getting Ahead

Head circumference is a very important measurement, and it is measured at each visit from birth to eighteen months of age. If possible, it's best to have the same doctor or nurse measure the head circumference at each visit for the greatest consistency and accuracy. This measurement denotes the ongoing growth of the bones of the skull and the developing brain. At this age, the fontanel is closing and the skull's suture lines are sealing. The skull and brain continue to grow.

The Brain

From the moment your pediatrician enters the examination room, he is examining your baby. Neurologic assessment goes way beyond the physical examination of the body. He is observing many things at once. Social interactions and responsiveness with parents and others are related to ongoing cognitive development. The appropriate use of all of the parts of the body is connected to her ongoing neuromuscular development.

Growth and Development

You are the proud parent of a one-year-old. You have watched him grow and develop for an entire year, and this has brought you and all of those around you great joy. By this age, your baby's gross motor development has probably included pulling to stand and cruising. Soon he will let go and balance unsteadily, eventually taking steps, beginning with a few from one anchor to another. Fine motor milestones should include holding toys or utensils well, having a good pincer grasp, self-feeding, and holding his cup or toothbrush. He should be able to place an object in a container, and he may turn pages in a book.

The development of speech, like all milestones, has a normal range, so refrain from comparing to others. He may or may not be using a word or two in context. He should be quite vocal, making his wishes clearly known with a variety of sounds. He may have a consistent yet indistinct utterance for a family pet or his sibling. By this age, you can easily differentiate the sounds for joy, sadness, and demands! Sounds become more meaningful.

He will surprise you with his intellectual development and the concepts he now grasps, from looking up when he hears an airplane to remembering to look for an object that was hidden and forgotten. He may begin to copy your sounds or moves, and he may move or bounce with music. He will begin to understand cause and effect.

In terms of social development, some babies are more reserved or outgoing than others, but he should be responsive and well related. If you feel connected, then there is little to worry about regarding significant developmental issues. React appropriately to his cues, and he will know that his thoughts and feelings are important to you.

Curious George

Your one-year-old is so aware of his surroundings now that it is amazing to you and your partner. He will be as curious as can be and will wish to investigate everything, not knowing if there is danger. All babies are different. Some are very cautious as they explore, and some just jump right in. Both are normal. Allow him to inquire, explore, and investigate safely. He will enjoy life this way without feeling hampered.

Off and Running

Gross motor development includes the stages from rolling to crawling to standing to walking. Once your baby has pulled to stand, he will cruise along, holding on to something or someone. He may walk while pushing a toy. Eventually he will let go and balance alone for a while, and then he will drop down and crawl again. Finally, he will take his first steps. The average age when this occurs is thirteen months.

Proud I Am

Your baby will show pride in his accomplishments as long as those around him acknowledge them. Positive reinforcement helps him develop healthy self-esteem, even at this age. Lavish praise upon him frequently. It is also not too early to set limits and teach him your invisible rules for your home and family, both for safety and behavior. Be firm, loving, and consistent as you teach him acceptable behavior versus unacceptable behavior.

Problem Solving

You will be amazed at the concepts your one-year-old appears to grasp at this young age, which you will see in the way he plays with certain toys, stacking, and the placement of puzzle pieces. He may look for, seek out, and find any dropped or hidden toys or objects (remember object permanence). He will play social games, remember things, and point with an index finger. He may follow simple commands.

Feeding

Most one-year-olds are eating machines by now, and they are growing as a result. Hopefully she is enjoying table food with you at mealtimes and making the transition from breast or bottle to the use of a cup. She should be able to hold her cup by herself! Her liquid diet should now include cow's milk and water. You can give her juice if firm stool or constipation is an issue, but otherwise it is best to avoid it. Juice can soften stool, but it is generally a source of empty calories.

Although more fluid is prudent in warmer climates or seasons, be careful that your baby doesn't drink so much that her appetite for solid foods decreases. This can lead to imbalanced nutrition and picky eating.

As far as solid foods are concerned, you are now able to give your baby any of your table foods, including berries, citrus fruits, and honey. Some pediatricians advise waiting until age two to introduce peanut-containing products. This is not always easy to do, especially if a sibling loves peanut butter! When you do introduce a peanut product, use a small amount in the morning so that you can monitor closely for any reactions, and have an anti-histamine available to use if needed. Call your doctor with any concerns.

There is currently an epidemic in our country known as childhood obesity. We must all be aware of the danger in order to prevent obesity in our babies. All infants differ in their makeup and metabolism. Some babies are more active than others, and some burn calories more effectively. You can prevent obesity by providing reasonable portions at meal-time, by offering healthy snacks, and by discouraging overeating.

Milk Magic

Now that your baby is one year old, she should be drinking whole milk as a part of her daily diet. Milk provides good nutrition, including protein, vitamin A, vitamin D, and calcium. Many overestimate the amount of dairy that infants and toddlers require daily. She should receive a total of eight to sixteen ounces of dairy daily. Remember that too much milk or fluid of any kind will decrease your baby's appetite for food, leading to nutritional imbalance.

Solidarity

Your baby has been receiving solids for many months now, enjoying them by spoon or by hand. You have probably offered a combination of jarred or homemade solids as well as your table food. Commercially prepared, higher-stage baby foods with more texture may still be used for convenience, but they are not needed. Table food in proper balance will provide the necessary nutrients for your one-year-old, and it is more cost-effective.

I Love to Eat

Mealtime should be fun and enjoyable, even if it is a messy business at the age of one! Allow a combination of fluids and solids, and remember to include all of the major food groups in a day. She may use utensils and her hands to self-feed, and you should still help her with the feeding exercise as needed. Most important, please be certain that the size is appropriate so that she does not choke. Avoid anything large or anything small and hard.

ALLERGIC REACTIONS

Siblings who are loving and helpful have good intentions, but be careful to watch them closely. Be certain not to allow big brother to share his snacks, which may be inappropriate in size or quality. This includes popcorn, nuts, or raisins. If allergic reactions to new foods occur, be prepared to recognize them, give an antihistamine, and call your pediatrician. Acute signs of food allergy may include fussiness, vomiting, local swelling of the lips, or hives on her skin (red, raised, itchy blotches).

Hot Shots

The recommended vaccines at twelve months of age include the first MMR and the fourth and last pneumococcal strep vaccine. A third injection that is recommended at this age is the PPD (purified protein derivative). The PPD is a skin test that is intended to determine if your baby has been exposed to an individual with active tuberculosis. It is not a vaccination against the infection, and it offers no protection. Positive reactions are rare, unless there has been direct exposure to someone with TB or if you and your baby have recently traveled to a country with an increased prevalence. The injection is given just under the skin of the forearm, and inspection for a reaction must be done by a nurse or doctor forty-eight to seventy-two hours later.

The pneumococcal strep vaccine is not new to your baby, as this is the fourth and final dose. This completes the series and protects him from invasive streptococcal infection. This streptococcus is one of the most common organisms that can cause middle ear infections, and less commonly can cause life-threatening infections such as pneumonia, meningitis, and bacteremia (infection in the bloodstream).

Finally, the first dose of MMR is recommended between twelve and fifteen months of age. This protects against three serious viral infections: measles, mumps, and rubella. The MMR vaccine has been a subject of controversy since 1998, when the medical journal *Lancet* published a research paper suggesting that the vaccine was associated with the development of autism. After much study, no established link has been found. The *Lancet* formally retracted the paper in 2010, citing fraudulent data and scandal related to its author.

I Need You

As with the injection at the nine-month well-baby visit, these vaccines will likely be given in the shoulder muscles. Hold your one-year-old close

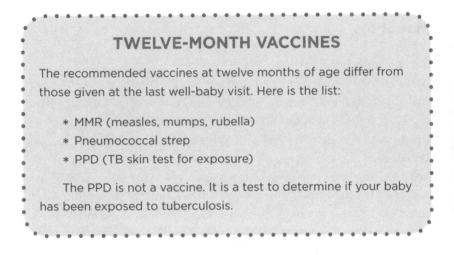

TWELVE-MONTH VACCINES

The recommended vaccines at twelve months of age differ from those given at the last well-baby visit. Here is the list:

* MMR (measles, mumps, rubella)
* Pneumococcal strep
* PPD (TB skin test for exposure)

The PPD is not a vaccine. It is a test to determine if your baby has been exposed to tuberculosis.

during the injections so that he will feel your comfort. At this age he will be keenly aware of what is happening, and it is normal for him to be afraid. After he receives the injections, walk around with him, talking, bouncing, hugging, and distracting him, and it will minimize the trauma.

Reaction Action

Adverse reactions to vaccines are uncommon, as you have witnessed over the past twelve months. If your baby has not reacted to the pneumococcal strep vaccine before, it is unlikely that he will now, although it is not impossible. Any vaccine may cause mild local swelling or tenderness, low-grade fever, and fussiness for a day. A small percentage of children will react to the MMR within one week, with fever and a noncontagious rash.

TB or Not TB

Tuberculosis skin testing is recommended at one year of age, even if you live in a low-risk area. High-risk areas include urban settings and countries in which the incidence of tuberculosis is increased. A PPD is placed just under the skin on your baby's forearm, and a bubble forms and recedes within an hour. This site must be inspected for any reaction in forty-eight to seventy-two hours. Positive reactions will be red and raised, resembling a large mosquito bite.

What's Next?

As you and your pediatrician review the twelve-month well-baby visit, reflect on the past year for a moment. You have loved, cared for, and nurtured your baby for one entire year, and it has taken a considerable amount of time and effort on your part, with or without the assistance of friends or family.

You have watched your baby grow, develop, and thrive during this year, and hopefully you have formed a close and trusted relationship with your pediatrician and his office staff as they watch over her with you. They are there to help, to answer questions, to calm your fears, and to guide you through any turbulent times that you may endure with your children. They have become part of your extended family, and most pediatricians and their staff feel honored by this.

At the close of this visit, your doctor will review any significant findings from the physical examination, and he will review your baby's growth using the growth charts for weight, length, and head circumference. He will also discuss your baby's dietary intake, confirming that her caloric intake has been adequate and that her diet is well balanced. This is not always easy as children begin to show preferences for taste and texture. Remember to maintain structure with a schedule, and seek to ensure a balanced diet with both fluids and solid foods. She should be enjoying whole milk, and she should be supplemented with a daily multivitamin and fluoride if your water supply is not fluorinated.

Make the transition from bottle to cup between nine and fifteen months of age, and you will not have to battle with a toddler later. This will also be better for dental health. Make tooth-brushing a positive part of her daily routine.

Bye-Bye, Baby

It is wonderful to watch your baby's ongoing development as she attains skills daily. She will enjoy pleasing you with each skill, and she will be thrilled with your praise and attention. Common thrill-inducers include waving hello or goodbye, clapping, playing peek-a-boo with you, and any other social game. Perhaps the most cherished and tender act is blowing kisses. She knows that this stands for mutual love and affection.

All Fall Down

Your one-year-old is mobile, and with mobility comes falling, and this often involves the head. Most trauma to the head is referred to as minor closed head trauma and does not result in significant head injury. Don't panic. Pick up your baby after a fall and console her in your arms, observing closely for any noticeable abnormality. If there is loss of consciousness, vomiting, lethargy, seizure, inconsolability, or inordinate swelling on the scalp, call your pediatrician immediately.

Final Questions

Your one-year-old is a walking (almost), talking (almost), unique individual with his own special personality, and you have seen this evolve steadily over the past year. At this age he is more mobile, prompting you to revisit safety concerns in his environment, both in your home and in the outside world in which he travels.

You can see gains not only in his gross motor development, but also in his fine motor development as he becomes adept at many tasks with each hand. Hand dominance may seem to be developing, but it is really too early to be certain.

You have seen that his speech and language development are progressing with receptive gains (what he hears and processes) and expressive gains (what you hear him say). Again, there is a normal range for each milestone, so please try not to compare him to siblings or friends. Rely on your pediatrician to address concerns with respect to a developmental delay in any area.

You have watched in awe as he has developed intellectually, gaining an understanding of concepts such as object permanence, and as he makes his needs and wants clearly known to you. Socially, he brightens your day and probably attracts the attention of others like a magnet. He will continue to thrive in a happy, healthy home where he can grow and develop with your care, your support, and your love. Keep up the good work!

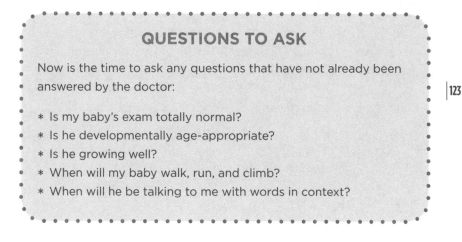

QUESTIONS TO ASK

Now is the time to ask any questions that have not already been answered by the doctor:

* Is my baby's exam totally normal?
* Is he developmentally age-appropriate?
* Is he growing well?
* When will my baby walk, run, and climb?
* When will he be talking to me with words in context?

Lefty or Righty

Parents often wonder whether their baby will be left-handed or right-handed, and you may be thinking about this. You may see some signs of hand dominance after your baby turns a year old, but this can be misleading. Most experts agree that consistent hand dominance develops between two and three years of age. Genetic factors play a significant role in hand dominance. There is no need to try to encourage right- or left-handedness.

Derma Trauma

As your baby passes his birthday, you will see him become more active than ever before, given normal motor development. His increased mobility brings with it increased danger to him and to his skin as he moves around. It is common to be bruised and scraped from falls as he learns to walk, coming in contact with various surfaces. Most minor abrasions and lacerations (scrapes and cuts) are best treated with topical antibiotic ointment to prevent skin infection.

Looking Ahead

Watch for many new signs of development by fifteen months of age. By that time, your little one will probably be walking, if not running, and trying to climb everything in sight. He should be saying at least three words in context, and he will be more responsive and reactive than ever. He may be blowing kisses, pointing to body parts, and following commands.

CHAPTER ELEVEN

Ill Visits and Emergencies

In addition to your newborn's regular wellness visits, he or she will likely encounter several mild illnesses during the first year of life that will require an ill visit to the doctor. It's helpful to know the signs and symptoms of minor illness, such as congestion and sleep disruption. It's especially important to recognize the signs of major illness, such as lethargy or inconsolability. We'll review both, as well as what to expect during a visit to the emergency room, including common tests and procedures, and how to prepare for a hospital stay.

When Should I Call My Pediatrician?

Most new parents are quite hesitant to call their pediatrician. You may feel this way now, but you need not. Part of the commitment a pediatric physician makes is to provide encouragement and education to mothers like you as she walks with you on this journey. During daily office hours most pediatricians hire and train nurses to handle most of the routine questions that arise. This allows you to receive answers to your questions so that the doctor can remain on schedule with patients—something you will appreciate when you are at the office for an appointment.

No question should be considered too small. Even if you are well read, you are expected to avail yourself of the expertise at your pediatric office. Your pediatrician will want you to feel comfortable calling with questions, even if only to confirm the validity of what you have read or have been told by friends or family. After office hours have passed, you may still call with questions. Although after-hours calls are technically for urgent needs, new parents might make after-hours calls until they gain more experience and confidence. Don't feel badly or think you are imposing. The on-call pediatrician is available at any hour. It is part of his or her commitment to you.

You are the best judge of your baby's behavior because you spend the most time with him. Your pediatrician will count on you to relay any information that may be helpful to her in assessing the baby's needs given the situation at hand. Remember to speak clearly and calmly when you call, and describe your baby accurately. Describe any changes in feeding, sleep pattern, temperature, and behavior in general.

Be Prepared
It is always wise to keep your important telephone numbers handy. Include your pediatrician's office phone number on this list. You may have the list on a bulletin board in your kitchen or office, or you may have a magnet on your refrigerator. In a true emergency, simply dial 911 and emergency service will be dispatched to your home or other location. Examples of a true emergency include seizure activity or an abrupt change in your baby's color or breathing pattern. These are rare entities.

Go to the Source
Routine medical advice is an important part of pediatric medicine. It is a part of everyday practice in a pediatric office. Pediatric nurses are trained to answer a broad range of questions that new and not-so-new moms have about their little ones. No question is regarded as too small or too silly. Feel free to call, especially if you are confused or uncertain.

The nurses know their limits. If they don't know the answer to your question, they will check with the doctor and then get back to you.

Stay Calm
Routine questions are one thing—don't hesitate to call with these—but call right away if you think your baby is sick. Try not to panic, even if

you are upset. Stay calm as you dial the doctor, and those around you will also remain calm. It's especially important to appear calm in the presence of your baby or any siblings, for they can easily sense your fear and anxiety. Remember, mom is considered right until proven otherwise. You know your baby better than anyone. Don't hesitate to call your pediatrician.

Pertinent Information

When you call your pediatrician's office with a medical concern, you should always give your baby's name, age, weight, medications (if any), allergies (if any), and any medical issues the baby has had to date. Then share the current concern, including her symptoms and their duration. Be prepared to share information with the nurse to whom you are speaking. This will allow her to be as helpful with her phone advice as possible. After hours, you may be speaking to a doctor who doesn't know your baby. He will also need to know this information in order to best address your concerns.

Whose Advice Is Best?

Today we are blessed with incredible technology and tremendous access to information on just about every subject. Most new moms have a computer and are well read. Perhaps you have been reading throughout your pregnancy in preparation for your baby and his or her care. Please be careful that you do not become overwhelmed as you read books or the Internet. You may be researching a particular subject, and you may be taken to the rarest of scenarios. This will not be helpful to you, as it can create confusion and induce anxiety. This is the last thing that you need as you are learning to care for your baby.

If you are uncertain about the information at hand, always feel free to check with your pediatrician and his staff. They are there to help, to reassure, and to educate. Whether the advice is from a book, the Internet, or a shared e-mail, you must seek to validate the information. You can always consult a website that is dedicated to evaluating urban legends, such as www.snopes.com. At this site one can choose a particular subject and do a search, and the site will deny or confirm validity of an e-mail posting whose message is suspect to you.

For the medical bottom line in pediatrics, consult the American Academy of Pediatrics. The academy is dedicated to the health of infants, children, and adolescents. The AAP website, www.aap.org, has a wealth of information. You can also consult the AAP book *Caring for Your Baby and Young Child, Birth to Age Five*. Two volumes follow—one for older children and one for adolescents. In general, books written by pediatricians who are fellows of the AAP can be trusted for their pediatric advice.

Well-Meaning Family

Wisdom comes with age. Your family members have much advice to offer you about your baby. Be a good listener, especially to the elderly, as they are not usually given the respect they deserve. Feel free to consult your baby's grandmother or aunt, and accept their advice graciously. However, beware of old wives' tales that have been handed down over time. Always feel free to check with your doctor and her staff to validate the information you receive.

Check in Anytime

You may hear breaking news on television about an infectious disease—check with your doctor. You may read in the newspaper about the latest breakthrough in infant care—check with your doctor. You may hear on the radio about a new controversy regarding vaccines for your baby—check with your doctor. You may read an alarming e-mail on the computer that applies to babies—check with your doctor.

Share the Information

Remember that you are not alone, and your partner also needs to be kept in the loop. Whenever either of you receive information regarding the care of your baby, it must be shared. Share the information you receive openly and accurately so that little is missed in the translation. When parents are on the same page with the same understanding, their baby's care will be optimized.

III Visits—Minor

During the first year of your baby's life, he will probably be affected by several mild illnesses. You will also notice changes in behavior. One of the most common causes for a change in your baby's behavior is teething. This is not an illness. Signs of teething may begin after two months of age, even though you may not see the teeth for many months. Symptoms of teething include drooling, fussiness, low-grade temperature elevation, rash, and loosened stool. When infants get infections, they are usually viral in origin, and they may display some of these same symptoms.

Additional signs and symptoms will alert you that he may have more going on than teething. For example, an upper respiratory infection (common cold) will yield increased nasal

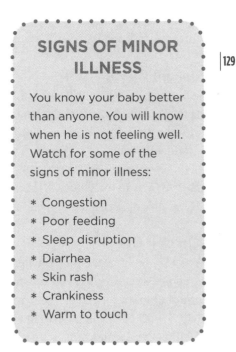

SIGNS OF MINOR ILLNESS

You know your baby better than anyone. You will know when he is not feeling well. Watch for some of the signs of minor illness:

* Congestion
* Poor feeding
* Sleep disruption
* Diarrhea
* Skin rash
* Crankiness
* Warm to touch

congestion with disrupted feeding and sleeping. If an ear infection ensues, your baby may cry while sucking due to pressure in the middle ear space. If a diaper rash is persistent and increasing, it may be more than the common diaper dermatitis; perhaps it is a yeast infection. If his stool pattern becomes very loose and diarrheal in nature without any dietary change, he may have a gastrointestinal virus, particularly if it is associated with vomiting and an elevated temperature. Always bring your baby to your pediatrician to be evaluated so that you can be confident in the diagnosis and the plan for your baby's care.

Thanks to moms, most babies don't have many illnesses during the first four to six months of life. Your baby receives your antibodies through the placenta, so she enjoys your immune system for those initial months until it dwindles, after which she must build her own immune system. It is then expected that she will endure frequent viral infections until two to three years of age.

Unhappy Baby

When baby's behavior is altered, she is trying to tell you that something is wrong. When she is clingy and fussy, she may be brewing an infection of some kind. This fussiness will go beyond the baseline fussiness in the infant with colic.

If your baby is warm to touch, this may also be a sign that she is beginning to fight an infection. Changes in behavior and low-grade temperature elevation can also be signs of teething, depending on the age of the baby.

Check It Out

You may be uncertain as to whether or not you need to have your baby seen and examined. This is normal. Rely on your knowledge of your baby and that inner feeling or "gut instinct." Don't hesitate to call your pediatrician's office to schedule an ill visit. You will be welcomed without judgment at the doctor's office. Your doctor and his staff are there to help.

Evaluation

At the doctor's office, your baby will stay in your loving arms for history taking. He may be weighed, and his temperature may be taken if he is in early infancy. Your pediatrician will examine the baby, looking closely for any physical findings that lead to a diagnosis. Once the exam is complete, the doctor will explain her impression, give a diagnosis, and discuss the plan of action.

Ill Visits—Major

Significant illnesses or life-threatening illnesses are rare in infants and children. However, you must be prepared to recognize the signs if they present themselves to you. The degree of change in your baby's behavior is much greater than during teething or a minor illness. Signs and symptoms of major illness in infancy are less subtle and more easily recognizable. A severe change in a baby's demeanor is one of the first signs— including either lethargy or inconsolability. Also, although a baby's skin can sometimes be temporarily mottled when bathing, this might otherwise be a sign of illness. A non-blanching rash with an appearance similar to broken blood vessels may be a sign of serious infection. Any kind of respiratory distress is cause for concern, including constant coughing, rapid breathing, audible

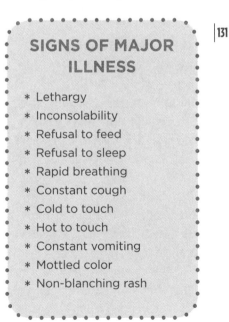

SIGNS OF MAJOR ILLNESS

* Lethargy
* Inconsolability
* Refusal to feed
* Refusal to sleep
* Rapid breathing
* Constant cough
* Cold to touch
* Hot to touch
* Constant vomiting
* Mottled color
* Non-blanching rash

wheezing, and retraction of the skin between the ribs with each breath, implying that the baby is working too hard.

Feeding may be difficult or refused by a sick infant. Feeding intolerance or constant vomiting is a concern, as dehydration can occur quickly in a baby, especially if it is associated with fever and watery stool. If any of these signs or symptoms of significant illness occur, please call your pediatrician right away. Early intervention is the best intervention.

Temperature elevation that occurs in a baby in the first two months of life could be a sign of serious infection. At this age a rectal temperature of 100.4 degrees Fahrenheit or greater prompts immediate evaluation, even in the absence of other symptoms. It could be the result of a mild reaction to an immunization or a response to a common viral infection, but it may be the first sign of a serious bacterial infection. Call for an evaluation right away.

132

Very Unhappy Baby

You will know right away if your baby has a very significant change in her usual behavior. A sick infant can be either lethargic or inconsolable despite your best efforts. Both the lethargic baby and the inconsolable baby will be difficult to feed. Do not try to force-feed, as they may choke. Pay close attention to your baby's skin tone and color. A baby who is very ill may display changes in her skin.

Check It Out

Signs of major illness in your baby must be reported to your pediatrician right away. You will be advised to have the baby seen and examined immediately.

During the day, he will probably be seen in your doctor's office. After office hours and through the night, the pediatrician may refer you to your local emergency room for evaluation.

Evaluation

Your baby will be weighed and her vital signs will be taken very carefully. These include her temperature, heart rate, respiratory rate, and blood pressure. Pulse oximetry may be done to measure oxygenation, especially if her breathing pattern is a concern. A pulse oximeter is a painless, lighted probe that is taped to a finger or toe to measure her ability to oxygenate. The pediatrician or emergency department physician will examine your baby thoroughly to determine the cause of her symptoms.

Testing 1, 2, 3

When a patient of any age is ill, tests may be required as part of the evaluation. Arriving at an accurate diagnosis is paramount if your baby is sick. When your baby is seriously ill, your pediatrician may recommend one or more tests in order to help make the diagnosis.

Testing involves procedures that have to be performed. Results of these tests, in combination with the findings on the baby's examination, will allow the doctor to fully assess the illness and arrive at the appropriate plan of treatment.

When serum values are needed, blood is drawn from a vein, or from an artery if necessary. This may take more than one attempt because infants' vessels are small. They may collapse, and they may not be as full when a baby is dehydrated.

When urine collection is required, urinary catheterization is used for the most accurate results. A small, sterile catheter is placed through the urethra to the bladder to collect the urine. The catheter is attached to a syringe into which the urine is aspirated. If oxygenation is in question, a pulse oximetry reading will be taken. This is performed by placing a painless probe on your baby's finger or toe. The probe takes the reading through the skin and yields a number.

Meningitis is an infection of the meninges, the covering of the brain and spinal cord. If your pediatrician wishes to rule out meningitis, a lumbar puncture (spinal tap) will be performed. A nurse holds the baby, and the doctor performs the procedure. Be assured that this is the easiest time and age to perform this procedure, as the anatomy is small and thin. No complication should be expected. It sounds frightening, but it is no greater in discomfort or risk than drawing blood.

All About the Holder

Proper holding is key when it comes to performing procedures to obtain specimens. Remain calm as you hold your baby, and follow the guidance of the technician, nurse, or doctor. It is best to hold lovingly but firmly, not allowing the fearful infant to be a moving target. Close attention to this will make the procedure more efficient and less traumatic for your baby.

PROCEDURES FOR TESTING

Many different modalities may be used for testing during your baby's evaluation. Some of these are associated with discomfort, and some of them are not:

* Venipuncture (blood drawing)
* Lumbar puncture (spinal tap)
* Bladder catheterization (urine removal)
* Imaging (ultrasound, X-rays, CT scans, or MRIs)
* Pulse oximetry (clip-on transducer on the finger or toe)

Clinical Expertise

Performing procedures to test a sick baby is both an art and a science. Trust that the person performing the procedure is qualified and has your baby's best interest at heart. A butterfly needle that is small enough for use on infants may be used to draw blood from a vein or an artery. A small spinal needle will be used between the vertebrae if a lumbar puncture is advised to rule out meningitis.

Send It Off

Once the specimens have been collected, console your baby. The procedures have been completed, and the discomfort will resolve shortly. The baby's specimens will be carefully handled and labeled. The specimens will then be sent to the lab for evaluation, and the results will be given to your doctor. This applies to the collection of urine, blood, stool, and spinal fluid. Imaging results are interpreted by a radiologist and reported directly.

Hospitalization

When babies are significantly ill, they may indeed need to be evaluated at the hospital. Always rely on the judgment of your pediatrician to guide you in this regard. She will know if the hospital is necessary to determine what is best for your little one. Perhaps an evaluation with testing is recommended, the results of which may determine the need for admission. The need for admission may be clear already. You may be referred to your local community hospital or to the nearest tertiary care center, again depending on the needs of your baby during this illness. Rest assured that you and the baby will be appropriately cared for in either setting with clinical expertise and compassion.

Plan ahead and pack personal items as if you may be staying, and you will be ahead of the game. Hospitals have plenty of diapers, wipes, formula, and food, so you won't need to worry about bringing any of those items. Occasionally a direct admission is arranged. More commonly, the initial evaluation occurs in the emergency department, and then your baby will be taken to the pediatric floor. There may be a delay while a room is prepared for you. The nursing staff will admit both of you and settle you into the room. The pediatrician will examine your baby, discuss the plan of treatment with you, and write orders for her care.

During the hospital stay, a pediatrician will attend to your baby daily. It may be your pediatrician, or it may be a pediatric hospitalist. A pediatric hospitalist is a board-certified pediatrician who has chosen to practice full time in a hospital setting. Pediatric hospitalists have special expertise in inpatient pediatric medicine. Their care can be fully trusted.

Going to the Hospital

A trip to the hospital may be recommended for you and your baby when your baby has a serious illness. Your pediatrician may wish to have testing done at the hospital, such as lab work and/or imaging in the radiology department. Depending on the test results and the baby's clinical status, admission to the hospital may be necessary. The initial evaluation and assessment will most likely take place in the emergency department.

Depending on where you live, hospitals may vary in size and scope. There are community hospitals and tertiary care centers. Some community hospitals have separate areas for pediatric patients, and some do not. They all have experience caring for children. Tertiary care centers are large regional hospitals that are teaching centers, usually associated with local schools of medicine. Tertiary care centers have pediatric emergency departments and inpatient wards for pediatric patients who require admission.

Checking In

If you are being sent to the hospital, bring supplies in case your baby is admitted to the inpatient ward. You might consider bringing a change of clothes for the baby, a change of clothes for yourself, and your toiletries. When you arrive at the hospital, check in at the emergency triage desk with your insurance information handy. You and your baby will be greeted warmly, and she will quickly be assessed to determine the degree of her illness.

Once your baby has been assessed, procedures for testing will ensue, and specimens will be sent off. If admission to the hospital is advised, you will be escorted from the emergency department to the pediatric ward. Most pediatric wards allow parents to room in with their children. They will make you feel comfortable during this stressful time. Rooming in is important for your baby at any age. He knows your voice, your smell, and your touch. Your presence will keep him feeling secure.

WHAT TO PACK FOR AN OVERNIGHT HOSPITAL VISIT

_____ Your baby's diaper bag (infancy)

_____ A change of clothes for your baby or child

_____ A change of clothes for yourself

_____ Your toiletries

_____ Your cellular phone

_____ Your baby's favorite toy, blanket, or stuffed animal

_____ Your love

RECORD OF ILLNESS, HOSPITALIZATION, ACCIDENT, OR INJURY

Date	Age	Illness/Hospitalization/Accident/Injury
_____	_____	_____
_____	_____	_____
_____	_____	_____
_____	_____	_____
_____	_____	_____
_____	_____	_____
_____	_____	_____
_____	_____	_____
_____	_____	_____
_____	_____	_____
_____	_____	_____
_____	_____	_____
_____	_____	_____
_____	_____	_____

CHAPTER TWELVE

Vaccines

Vaccines and their administration have been under scrutiny for the past decade, in particular with respect to suspicions regarding their efficacy and their potential adverse effects. Vaccination has long been a highly charged subject. Despite the controversy, anyone who looks at the history of vaccinations will be amazed. Long before the advent of big business and pharmaceutical companies, many individuals dedicated their lives to the research and development of vaccines. Their goal has always been to produce safe and effective protection from vaccine-preventable diseases.

Many years of study have been devoted to reducing infection and death in children and adults, and these efforts continue today. The first vaccinations can be traced back to 1798, with efforts to prevent smallpox. In the late 1800s, rabies and the plague were targeted. After the turn of the twentieth century, the war against disease continued with even greater devotion and strength, and vaccines were produced for many organisms whose names you will recognize. These include cholera, typhoid, diphtheria, pertussis, tetanus, tuberculosis, yellow fever, and influenza. Beginning in the mid-1900s, vaccinations were successfully produced to protect against polio, measles, mumps, rubella, anthrax, meningococcus, hepatitis B, HIB (Hemophilus influenzae B), varicella (chicken pox), rotavirus, and streptococcus pneumoniae.

Your pediatrician relies on the vaccine recommendations of the American Academy of Pediatrics Committee on Infectious Diseases. This committee is comprised of pediatric infectious disease specialists—pediatricians who have added to their general pediatric specialty training with fellowships in pediatric infectious disease. They endorse the work of the National Vaccine Advisory Committee, and they collaborate with the Centers for Disease Control (CDC).

A History of Vaccines

The term *variolation* describes the process that has led to the success of vaccinations in public health today. If a healthy host is exposed to material from an infected host, the healthy host will develop its own protective antibodies. In 1796, Dr. Edward Jenner inoculated a boy with cowpox fluid and later exposed him to smallpox without a resulting infection. Dr. Jenner then coined the term *vaccine,* using the word *vaca,* which comes from the Latin word for *cow.*

Smallpox was at one time a most devastating infection, causing many to be ill and die during outbreaks. Years after Jenner's work, the FDA licensed a vaccine made from the "New York City Board of Health" strain. The last outbreak in the United States occurred in 1949, and the last known case occurred in Somalia in 1977. Routine smallpox vaccination stopped in 1971, and the World Health Assembly declared the world free of smallpox in 1980.

Rabies virus was fatal in all affected individuals until the advent of post-exposure prophylaxis with vaccine. This virus is transmitted by infected animals and causes encephalitis, an inflammation of the brain. The rabies vaccine was harvested from infected rabbits by Louis Pasteur and Emile Roux in 1885. After one has been exposed to rabies virus, receiving rabies immune globulin and rabies vaccines is protective.

Some bacterial or viral infections have available vaccines that do not enjoy widespread use. Cholera is one of them. Vibrio Cholerae is a bacteria that can affect the small bowel, causing severe vomiting, diarrhea, and dehydration. Infection is contracted after exposure to contaminated food or water, and the diagnosis is confirmed by stool culture. Prevention relies on proper sanitation practices. An oral vaccine is available, but the CDC does not recommend its prophylactic use.

Math Is Life

When you consider the numbers, you can see just how valuable vaccinations have been. It has not been that long since many were stricken with disease and death from infection throughout the world. For centuries there was no protection from pandemics and epidemics. This is not the case today. Your baby's future is bright with respect to preventable infection. There are individuals alive today who remember their friends and loved ones being afflicted by deformity and paralysis as a result of poliovirus.

Since the licensing of polio vaccine in the mid-1950s, this virus has been all but eradicated in the United States. Rubella, or German measles, is a virus that can affect a fetus during the first trimester if an expectant mother in infected. In the mid-1960s thousands were born with birth defects as a result of a rubella epidemic.

Also, prior to the vaccine era, measles caused death and destruction to families when the disease was epidemic. It is no longer an active issue because of the efficacy of the vaccine. Hemophilus influenzae type B (HIB) can cause life-threatening epiglottitis, an infection of the epiglottis in the throat, and it can cause meningitis, but this has hardly been seen in the last twenty years. Varicella, or chicken pox, once claimed almost one hundred lives per year prior to routine immunization.

All of these are stunning reductions in the number of infections and their aftereffects, including deaths, and they can all be attributed to the success of vaccines. Public health has improved, there is less damage to individuals and families, and life spans are much longer. Indeed, the physicians who are in training today will most likely never see patients with many of these infections. They may simply have to read about them in their textbooks, or they may just have to ask some of us old fellows what it was like to see those infections and the suffering they caused.

Do the Math

The number of infectious diseases in existence today—and their fallout—does not compare with those that existed many years ago. Poliovirus is a prime example of this. Active vaccination began after the vaccine was licensed in the United States in 1962. Since that time, the oral vaccine prevented most cases, with the exception of wildvirus, which could be associated with the live oral vaccination. At present, only the inactivated (injected) vaccine is used, and poliovirus is all but eradicated in our country.

History Lesson

The first generation of vaccines formally began in 1798 with Dr. Edward Jenner's smallpox vaccine. This period continued until 1945 when the first vaccine against influenza virus began to be used. The second generation of vaccines began in the 1950s and has seen the production and use of more than twenty vaccines. Math is indeed life, as the number of cases of infectious diseases, with their damage and death, has been severely reduced over time.

Combination Platter

Mumps, measles, and rubella are very virulent viruses that can cause serious illness or death. Measles vaccine was first licensed in 1963, mumps vaccine was licensed in 1967, and rubella vaccine was licensed in 1969. The number of infections from these three viruses dropped as a result of the active vaccination campaign against them. A combination vaccine uniting the three vaccines was licensed in the United States in 1971.

Influenza

Influenza is a potent virus that still causes many infections and deaths per year around the world. Use of influenza vaccine began in 1945, with the current vaccine licensed in 1978. It is safe and effective. Swine flu pandemics occurred in 1976 and again in 2010 (H1N1), prompting widespread vaccination to fight it. Two new proteins have been added to the yearly influenza vaccine in order to prevent the new H1N1 influenza infection.

Preservatives

There has been a great deal of controversy over the use of preservatives in the production of vaccines, particularly the vaccines that have been so successfully used in our children. Preservatives were actively used for many years in multi-dose vials of vaccination, sometimes with ten or more doses contained in one vial. Considering the number of vacci- | 143
nations in the recommended childhood schedule, this amounted to a lot of exposure. The most commonly used preservative was thiomersal, an organomercury compound known for its antiseptic and antifungal qualities. You may know this as thimerosal, the common spelling used in the United States. It was once thought that elevated levels of mercury resulting from this preservative may have caused neurodevelopmental maladies. In addition, some thought that this may have been partially responsible for the rise in the number of children diagnosed as being on the autistic spectrum. This speculation led the American Academy of Pediatrics and the Centers for Disease Control to request the removal of the preservative from vaccines as a precautionary measure.

All of the vaccines that your baby will receive are now single-dose, preservative-free vaccines. This has been the case since the year 2000. They are safe for your baby and effective in preventing infectious diseases. More than eight studies have been conducted in as many years to see if the rate of autism has decreased since the removal of preservatives from childhood vaccines, and the numbers have not changed.

As of yet, there has been no proof of causality between vaccines and their past preservatives and neurodevelopmental abnormalities. Ongoing research has and will continue to try to delineate a cause for the rise in these issues in our children. Pediatricians are dedicated to preventing suffering, and we are open and willing to listen to any theory on the subject.

Thiomersal

There is a trace of thiomersal in the influenza vaccine that is available for individuals who are two years of age and older. Again, thiomersal is an organomercury compound that can cause an elevated mercury level in children. In the ten years since the removal of thiomersal from vaccines, the number of diagnoses of autism has not decreased. Some parents have chosen to use chelation therapy (the removal of heavy metals) for children who are on the autistic spectrum based on their exposure to thiomersal. This is not routinely recommended, and it is not without risk. Results have not been conclusive to show uniformly significant results in improvement.

Additives

Additives have also been used in addition to preservatives in the manufacture of vaccines. Some vaccines may contain formaldehyde in small, harmless amounts to eliminate harmful effects of bacterial toxins in the vaccine. Some vaccines are live virus vaccines. Human serum albumin is an additive that stabilizes the live virus. Rest assured that the small amount of additives has been deemed safe for your baby based on all of our research.

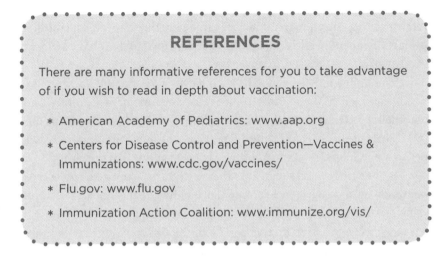

REFERENCES

There are many informative references for you to take advantage of if you wish to read in depth about vaccination:

* American Academy of Pediatrics: www.aap.org

* Centers for Disease Control and Prevention—Vaccines & Immunizations: www.cdc.gov/vaccines/

* Flu.gov: www.flu.gov

* Immunization Action Coalition: www.immunize.org/vis/

DTAP, HIB, and Pneumococcal Strep

DTAP, HIB, and pneumococcal strep are three bacterial vaccines your baby will receive in her first year of life. The vaccination schedule recommended by the American Academy of Pediatrics includes sequential vaccination against many vaccine-preventable viruses and bacteria. Let's look a bit more in depth at each vaccine your baby will receive.

The DTAP is actually three vaccines in one, and each one protects against a different bacteria. Diphtheria can cause severe mouth and throat infections, swollen glands, and pneumonia. The vaccine contains a toxoid that induces immunity to the diphtheria toxin. Tetanus can cause severe muscle contractions, and it is transmitted through any break in the skin, most easily via a puncture wound (hence the "rusty nail" warning). This vaccine also contains a toxoid protecting against the toxin. Pertussis, or whooping cough, can cause a serious pneumonia that requires hospitalization in infancy. It can be life threatening. The vaccine protects against the bacteria, and its acellular formulation has been free of adverse effects for over fifteen years.

Hemophilus influenzae B (HIB) is a bacteria, despite the fact that the word *influenza* is in the name. HIB can cause pneumonia, epiglottitis, and meningitis. Fifteen years ago, it was the leading cause of meningitis in children. Since the use of the vaccine, there have been only a few hundred cases per year as opposed to twenty thousand cases resulting in many deaths.

The pneumococcal conjugate vaccine protects against streptococcus pneumoniae, a serious form of strep that can invade the bloodstream and cause life-threatening sepsis, pneumonia, or meningitis. This is a different strep from the strep on the skin or in the throat. Even with the vaccine and a decreased number of infections, this strep takes the lives of one to two hundred children annually. Since 2000, the conjugate vaccine has worked well to prevent infection in babies. Prior to 2000, a polysaccharide vaccine was available, but it wasn't very effective. Infants and the elderly both receive a vaccine to protect them against this strep, as they are the most vulnerable to the infection.

DTAP

This vaccine protects against diphtheria, tetanus, and pertussis. Each of these organisms is a bacteria that can cause significant infection and can even be life threatening in infancy. In the past, the pertussis portion was made using the whole cell technique, utilizing the entire organism, and the DTAP vaccine caused high fever and fussiness for a day or two. Today the pertussis portion is made using the acellular technique, utilizing only the necessary part of the organism, resulting in few or no adverse effects.

Pertussis

Bordatella pertussis is the name of the organism that causes whooping cough, an infection that is especially dangerous to your baby. This bacterial infection causes paroxysms of harsh, prolonged staccato coughing that may last for many days. The repetitive episodes of coughing may end in gagging, vomiting, or gasping air back in, which is called the whoop. The incidence of pertussis is low, but when babies have this infection, they usually need to be admitted to the hospital.

Hemophilus Influenzae B

HIB is a bacteria that can cause life-threatening infection, in particular meningitis in infants. In the past, this bacteria caused infection in thousands of infants, resulting in damage to their bodies or death. Epiglottitis was a common result of infection, causing a red, swollen epiglottis, which threatened the infant airway. Since the advent and widespread use of the HIB vaccine, these infections are almost a thing of the past.

Streptococcus Pneumoniae

Invasive streptococcal infections are no longer common, but they still occur and they can be life threatening. Streptococcus pneumoniae is unlike group A strep of the throat or the strep that affects the skin. It is invasive and can invade the bloodstream, causing sepsis. Sepsis is a bacterial infection in the bloodstream, which can be life threatening.

Babies who have this infection require hospitalization, intravenous antibiotics, and supportive care in order to survive. Since the year 2000, the pneumococcal conjugate vaccine has greatly decreased the incidence of this disease.

IPV, HBV, and Rotavirus

IPV, HBV, and rotavirus are three anti-viral vaccines your baby will receive during his first year of life. Vaccination against viral infections is just as important as protection against bacterial infections. Viruses can also cause serious infection in your baby, and they can even be life threatening under the right circumstances. Never underestimate the power of a virus.

Poliovirus can cause paralysis. It crippled thousands each year, prior to the 1950s. In 1916 six thousand people died, and more than twenty-five thousand were paralyzed. OPV, or oral polio vaccine, is a live viral vaccine, and IPV, or inactivated polio vaccine, is a killed vaccine—the only one used today in the United States.

Hepatitis B is a virus that causes inflammation of the liver and, though rare, poses the potential for liver failure. Its transmission is through infected blood or sexual contact with intimate secretions. Unless you are positive for hepatitis B, your baby is not at high risk. Still, three doses of the HBV vaccine are recommended by eighteen months of age. The vaccinations are quite safe, with little or no adverse effects. Liver failure is an uncommon occurrence with hepatitis B infection, but it is uniformly fatal. Liver transplants have not been successful.

Rotavirus is a virulent virus that can affect your baby's gastrointestinal tract. The infection caused by this virus results in vomiting and diarrhea. Combined with fever, fluid loss can easily cause an infant to become dehydrated. Rotavirus is the leading cause of these symptoms in childhood, and it is especially dangerous to your baby in his first twelve months. A rotaviral infection will prompt hospital admission for intravenous hydration until symptoms have resolved. Two or three oral doses of the rotavirus vaccine are given, depending on which of the two brands is used. Both are safe and effective to confer immunity against rotavirus.

Thanks to the dedication that parents have had in following the recommended vaccine schedule for their infants and children, all three of these significant viral infections are uncommon.

Poliovirus
Poliovirus is almost a thing of the past now that the incidence rate is the lowest it has ever been. Inactivated polio vaccine was licensed in 1955, and

the elimination of polio was certified in the Americas in 1994. Oral polio vaccine is a live viral vaccine, and it is still used in other countries. Inactivated polio vaccine is a killed viral vaccine given by injection, and it is the only type used in the United States.

Hepatitis B

Hepa means "liver," and the suffix *-itis* means "inflammation," so any type of hepatitis affects the function of the liver. Hepatitis infections have different modes of transmission. Hepatitis B is transmitted by blood and sexual contact. Hepatitis A is transmitted by the fecal-oral route. And hepatitis C is secondary to needle sharing. In extreme cases, this infection can cause liver failure, for which there is no curative treatment.

Three doses of the HBV vaccination will protect against hepatitis B infection, and they are given by eighteen months of life. If you are positive for hepatitis B, your baby should receive an earlier schedule for these three vaccines. The recommendation is for vaccination in infancy, even though most babies are not at high risk. The HBV vaccines are safe and effective to confer immunity with little or no adverse effect.

|149

Rotavirus

Many different viruses can affect your baby's GI tract, but this virus causes a particularly serious infection. Fever, vomiting, and a large volume of diarrheal stool can quickly lead to dehydration in infants. Stool can be cultured to confirm the otherwise clinical diagnosis, and hydration is the hallmark of therapy for the baby. Is it not unusual for your baby to require hospital admission for intravenous hydration to remain safe.

Varicella and the PPD

By the time your baby has reached her first birthday, she will have received many immunizations. You can be proud of the commitment that you have made to keep her safe in this life in every way, including protecting her from vaccine-preventable infectious diseases. You, your family, and your pediatrician have formed the team that is determined to protect her from any suffering. The next vaccine that she will likely receive is the one that can prevent the chicken pox, or varicella. Prior to the advent of the vaccine, more than four million individuals—mostly children—were affected in the United States, and there were close to one hundred deaths per year from complications. The numbers continue to decrease.

The varicella vaccine was licensed in 1995 for use in the United States, but it has been used in other countries, such as Japan, for a longer period of time. The vaccine has been administered to tens of thousands of children, and it has not been associated with any controversy with regard to significant adverse effects. It is a live virus vaccine, which is kept frozen until it is used. Varicella is caused by the zoster virus, and it can cause fever, malaise, and itchy blisters (pox) almost anywhere on the body, including the skin and mucous membranes.

Varicella

Chicken pox is caused by the varicella-zoster virus, a herpes virus known as human herpes virus type 3. Varicella-zoster virus, or VZV, is one of eight herpes viruses that affect humans, and it is the same virus that causes shingles in adults.

More than 90 percent of children now receive the varicella vaccine, which is administered between twelve and fifteen months of age. In 2007 a second dose was recommended at four years of age to ensure immunity in the school-age years.

Pox in Your Socks

Chicken pox occurs on the trunk, then spreads centrifugally (outward) to the face, scalp, arms, and legs. Chicken pox can also be found in the mucous membranes of the mouth and throat, the nose, and the vagina.

Complications of chicken pox have included life-threatening infection, such as pneumonia, meningitis, and brain abscess. Chicken pox parties to share the infection and develop immunity are not advisable; it is best to receive the vaccine.

Varicella Vibe

The varicella vaccine has been proven both safe and effective over many years. A small percentage of children will get a few pox on their skin two to three weeks after receiving the vaccine. This is a mild adverse effect of the vaccine that is not at all medically significant for the vaccine recipient. If she does have any vaccine-related pox, she is contagious to others until they have dried up and resolved.

Tuberculosis

PPD stands for "purified protein derivative," the standard skin test to determine exposure to tuberculosis. Your baby is at low risk unless she has been exposed to someone with active TB or has traveled to a country in which TB is endemic. PPD is the TB skin test, whereas the BCG (Bacilli Calmette-Guerin) is a vaccine to prevent tuberculosis. BCG is not recommended for use in the United States because of our low risk for TB and because of its interference with TB skin-testing reactivity.

IMMUNIZATION RECORD

Vaccine	Date	Doctor
Hepatitis B (HBV)	_____	_____
Rotavirus	_____	_____
Diptheria, Tetanus, Pertussis (DTAP)	_____	_____
Hemophilus Influenzae type B (HIB)	_____	_____
Pneumococcal Strep	_____	_____
Inactivated Poliovirus (IPV)	_____	_____
Influenza	_____	_____
Measles, Mumps, Rubella (MMR)	_____	_____
Varicella	_____	_____
Hepatitis A (HAV)	_____	_____
Meningococcal	_____	_____

Notes: _____

_____

_____

_____

CHAPTER THIRTEEN

Common Infections

Newborns often get infections just like adults, but it can be frightening when you're a new parent. This chapter will cover everything from colds, thrush, diaper rash, conjunctivitis, ear infections, group B strep, rotavirus, roseola, meningitis, and much more. It will outline the symptoms to look for, how you can make your newborn more comfortable if he or she does get one of these infections, and what types of treatment options are available.

The Cold (aka URI)

One of the most common infections to affect your baby is the upper respiratory infection, or URI. This is simply the technical term for the common cold. A cold comes from one of many viruses that travel through the air by droplet. These viruses are airborne and are easily transmitted from one host to another. Your baby will be exposed to airborne viruses almost everywhere he goes. Please don't let this inhibit your activity, as most viral infections are more annoying than they are significant or dangerous.

If you or your partner have a cold, your baby may be exposed to a respiratory virus in your home. If he has a sibling, your baby will undoubtedly share some of these common infections. It's impractical to try to separate siblings. They live and love in the same home, and these viruses are airborne. Of course, it is prudent to encourage good hand-washing and hygiene in your home in order to prevent the spread of infection. Your baby will also be exposed when out and about in the community. When he has a cold, he may have a low-grade fever, nasal congestion, and a cough.

TAKING YOUR BABY'S TEMP

BOTTOMS UP

The true core temperature is obtained by taking the temperature with a rectal thermometer. Infection may cause your baby to have a higher or a lower temperature than she usually has. This is called hyperthermia or hypothermia, and either should prompt a visit to the pediatrician for evaluation. If your baby has an increased or a decreased temperature, it may be a sign that she is fighting an infection.

THUNDER UNDER ARM

Another acceptable way to take a temperature in infants is the axillary, or underarm, temperature measurement. Simply place the thermometer under the arm, and hold the arm to her side gently so the arm cannot move. Add a point to the number that you receive, and this will be the same reading as if you had taken it rectally. Your pediatrician will examine your baby to determine if there is infection, what type, and the plan of action to follow.

This will be associated with a decrease in appetite and sleep disruption. Infants breathe out of their noses when they are feeding, so nasal congestion will make him quite unhappy.

In infancy, the first signs of infection are generally the alteration of feeding and sleeping. These will vary from his usual routine, most often with less of each. Due to nasal congestion, he may stop and start as he drinks. On occasion, an infant with a respiratory infection will sleep more, but more often his sleep is broken up, again due to congestion. The color of his nasal secretions is not that important. It may be clear or cloudy.

Moisten the Air

Use a cool-mist humidifier when he is sleeping, and keep him at an angle in the crib with his head elevated. The humidifier allows him to breathe in moistened air so that his secretions won't dry up and make him even more uncomfortable. Elevation of the head will help with drainage. You can adjust his crib so that his head is higher, providing a slight angle. Your humidifier should be close to the crib. If it is across the room, it will not be effective to moisten the air he breathes.

Use a Nasal Bulb Syringe

Babies need clear nasal passages to breathe comfortably during feedings. You can achieve this with a nasal bulb syringe. Squeeze the bulb, then insert the syringe into the nostril far enough to create a seal, and then release the bulb to suction. Your baby will not like having a cold, and he will really dislike his nasal secretions being suctioned out. Continue to suction periodically as needed despite this. You are helping him! If secretions are dry, use a few saline (saltwater) drops in each nostril prior to using the suction bulb.

Beyond the Cold

The treatment for a cold is not complicated. Cold medications should not be used during this first year of life. It's important to recognize signs and symptoms of more significant infection. If these occur, consult your pediatrician. If your baby has an audible wheeze, cough, or rapid breathing, or if he seems lethargic, inconsolable, or refuses to feed at all, he must be seen and examined by your doctor immediately.

Bronchiolitis

You have read about the common cold, and perhaps your baby has already experienced one. The cold, or URI, is more annoying to her than it is dangerous. Bronchiolitis is more significant. Bronchiolitis is a condition that can occur in the first one to two years of life, more often during the winter months. It is caused by a respiratory virus and leads to inflammation of the bronchioles, the smallest airways in your baby's lungs. Like the upper respiratory "cold," this condition is also viral, not bacterial, and it includes congestion, sneezing, fever, and fussiness.

The baby with bronchiolitis will also cough, wheeze, and breathe rapidly, and she will have to work harder than usual to breathe. As a result, you may see retractions of the skin between her ribs. She will show a significant decrease in appetite and an increase in sleep disruption as a result of her efforts to breathe. Nasal congestion and secretions can be more copious than during the common cold. Although bronchiolitis can be caused by one of many viruses, the most commonly implicated culprit is RSV, or respiratory syncytial virus. The diagnosis is made clinically (by examination), but your pediatrician may order a chest X-ray or a nasal washing to culture for RSV.

The treatment of bronchiolitis is basically supportive, with the clearing of nasal secretions and humidified air from a vaporizer, and maintaining good hydration with her usual intake of fluids. If your baby has too much trouble breathing, your pediatrician may recommend that she be admitted to the hospital for monitoring and for concentrated humidity in a tent with a bit of supplemental oxygen. Bronchodilator medication may be used, particularly if there is a family history of asthma, as the physiologic process is similar.

IT'S A MYTH!

Fever has been a source of great fear and concern for parents for many years. Pediatricians are often asked by new parents how high a temperature has to be before they should rush to the nearest hospital's emergency department. The truth is that fever is your friend. It is counterintuitive, but the infant, child, or adult with a normal, healthy immune system is able to mount a fever as a defense mechanism. It is one of the ways that your body fights for itself.

When infection occurs, most of us have an elevation in temperature known as fever. The real concern with fever is the rate of change. A rapid rise or fall in temperature can induce a seizure, sometimes called a febrile fit or febrile seizure. It's not the number that we reach but the rapid pace at which temperature moves that can induce a seizure. However, in the first two months of age, infants are especially at risk for significant infection, either viral or bacterial. If your baby has a rectal temperature of 100.4 degrees Fahrenheit or higher, she should be seen immediately by your pediatrician. At this age the number is meaningful, and it impacts the plan of treatment.

Testing 1, 2, 3

When a baby has bronchiolitis and has to work harder to breathe, she compensates by breathing more rapidly than usual. Even though she has an increased respiratory rate, she still may not be receiving an adequate amount of oxygen with each breath. In the pediatric office or at your hospital, her oxygenation can be measured easily and painlessly. A pulse oximeter is attached to her finger or toe to give a numerical measurement of her ability to oxygenate.

Warning Signs

Bronchiolitis is not as common as a simple cold, and you must be able to recognize the signs and symptoms. Cold symptoms such as congestion, decreased appetite, altered sleeping pattern, fussiness, and temperature elevation all occur. A frequent, "tight-sounding" hacking cough and audible wheezing ensue. A wheeze is a fine, high-pitched whistling noise, usually as she breathes out (exhale phase). If these conditions worsen, she may breathe rapidly and have retractions of the skin between her ribs with each labored breath.

Thrush

Thrush is a common infection that can affect your baby in many ways. It is another infection that can be annoying and uncomfortable, but it is not dangerous or life threatening. Thrush, or candidiasis, is caused by a yeast organism known as candida albicans. Yeast organisms thrive in moist environments. We have yeast as part of our normal flora, and it is kept at bay by our normal bacterial flora. When we are taking an antibiotic, the normal bacterial flora are depleted, and yeast can then overgrow, causing a yeast infection. Yeast growth increases whenever there is a warm, moist environment. It is the same organism that can cause a yeast infection, or vaginitis, in a woman. Moist environments that are attractive to yeast include the mouth, the vagina, and the skin in the diaper environment.

Your baby may even get a yeast infection in his mouth without being on an antibiotic. He may get it from your nipple and areola, or he may get it from the rubber from a bottle or pacifier. Yeast grows rapidly without either of you knowing it, and all of a sudden he is unhappy with symptoms. The symptoms of thrush, or oral candidiasis, include white patches or plaques on his buccal mucosa, gingival surfaces, and tongue. The buccal mucosae are the moist inner surfaces of the cheeks, and the gingivae are his gums. These white patches don't gently scrape off like residual milk will. If the patches go unnoticed and become thickened, they will be uncomfortable for your baby, leading to poor feeding with decreased frequency and amounts. If your baby is feeding poorly and has altered his usual pattern, look closely for white patches when he yawns or cries.

You can prevent yeast infections by following a few simple steps. If you are breast-feeding, gently cleanse your nipple and areola area with warm soap and water on a regular basis, drying thoroughly. Wash bottle nipple assemblies and pacifiers with soap and hot water and thoroughly dry between assembly parts where moisture will collect. This will prevent the yeast from growing.

If you suspect that your baby has a yeast infection, bring him to your pediatrician for evaluation. Yeast infections are treated with a specific medication that is available by prescription. Antifungal medications are placed into the baby's mouth by dropper one or more times daily, depending on the medication. Place the medication into his mouth after a feeding so that it will not be washed away immediately.

Monilial Dermatitis

Most babies will develop irritated skin in the diaper area during their first year of life. Your baby's skin is sensitive, and it can react to different stimuli and become inflamed. Some babies never get a diaper rash, but most will at some point.

The perianal skin (around the anus) of the newborn and the skin of the buttocks are not used to frequent exposure to urine and stool. This was not an issue for the fetal skin when it was always moist in utero. Even the best-kept babies may react to such exposure by becoming inflamed. The common diaper dermatitis appears as a chafing. It can be quite uncomfortable for your baby, and it is best treated with a thick barrier at each diaper change, so that it will heal while being protected from the next exposure. Almost any emollient will do. Be certain to use generous amounts!

The common diaper rash is not infectious. Infection can indeed occur in this area, and it can be fungal. Yeast dermatitis is fungal, and it has a typical appearance. Also known as monilial dermatitis, it is often associated with thrush, the yeast infection that can occur in a baby's mouth. It can simply pass through the GI tract and affect the perianal skin and the buttocks. It is typically a deeper red, and it can be seen in the folds of the groin. Its classic feature is satellite lesions. These are tiny red dots that appear at the periphery of the rash as it spreads. They are flat red dots that you may see all around the edges of the rash. The other hallmark is that this rash will not resolve with the standard diaper creams or ointment that you use for typical diaper rashes. This dermatitis persists until it is treated with an antifungal medication.

What Is Up Often Goes Down

Thrush occurs in the mouth, which is the beginning of a tube within a tube. That is, the GI tract goes from the mouth to the anus. Yeast that is in the mouth can naturally travel through the GI tract to the anus and out onto the skin.

If yeast reaches the perianal skin and buttocks, babies can develop a yeast infection of the skin. If a yeast infection occurs and goes untreated, it will continue to spread and can become quite painful.

Yeast Overgrowth

Yeast infections are common fungal infections that can affect the mucous membranes of both the mouth and the skin. Yeast growth occurs in warm, moist areas, such as in a diaper, which, by definition, is a good incubator. If a broad-spectrum antibiotic is needed for a bacterial infection, all bacterial flora are reduced in your baby's body. Less-healthy bacteria can lead to an overgrowth of yeast, which in turn causes the yeast infection on her skin.

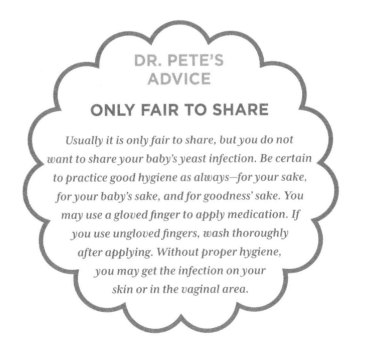

DR. PETE'S ADVICE

ONLY FAIR TO SHARE

Usually it is only fair to share, but you do not want to share your baby's yeast infection. Be certain to practice good hygiene as always—for your sake, for your baby's sake, and for goodness' sake. You may use a gloved finger to apply medication. If you use ungloved fingers, wash thoroughly after applying. Without proper hygiene, you may get the infection on your skin or in the vaginal area.

Top That

Any irritation of your baby's skin must be treated with applications of topical cream or ointment for her comfort and safety. Typical diaper rash is covered with a thick, non-medicinal barrier so that the inflammation will resolve simply with frequent protection. Fungal skin infections require an antifungal cream or ointment to adequately treat the infection. Antifungal medications are available over the counter or by prescription. Your pediatrician will determine what is necessary for treatment.

Conjunctivitis

Conjunctivitis, or "pink eye," is a common entity in infants and children. This word comes from *conjunctiva*, the lining of the sclera (white part of the eye) and the eyelids. The suffix *-itis* means "inflamed." Conjunctivitis is an inflammation of this lining, and it can be caused by allergy or infection. Allergic conjunctivitis usually happens during the months when pollen is flying about, and it is rarely seen in infancy. This type of inflammation generally occurs in both eyes, is quite itchy, and is without discharge.

Infection can also cause conjunctivitis in your baby, and it can be either viral or bacterial. The more common cause would be a virus, with obvious inflammation of the white part of the eye and the eyelid linings. The virus can be present in one or both eyes, and it will be irritating to her. This will cause her to be fussy, and it can affect feeding and sleeping patterns. Fever is not associated with conjunctivitis, unless there are other simultaneous infections.

Unfortunately, there is no rule stating that your baby can't have more than one cause for complaint. She may be teething, have a cold, and have pink eye all at the same time! A viral conjunctivitis should resolve without medication, but it can take many days to do so.

Bacteria can also cause pink eye. A bacterial conjunctivitis will usually make itself known by causing a discharge from one or both eyes, and this will be irritating to your baby as well. She may awaken with one or both eyelids sticking together. The discharge is yellow or green and is mucopurulent (containing mucous or pus). Broad-spectrum antibiotic drops are used to fight bacterial conjunctivitis. Treatment is based on clinical examination. Unless there are complications, scrapings for cultures are not routinely done, and referrals to specialists are not usually necessary.

Eye See You
Your pediatrician examines your baby's eyes with a special instrument called an ophthalmoscope. Conjunctivitis can be an allergic response to the environment or a given season, such as when pollen occurs in the spring. Allergic conjunctivitis can occur in infants, but it is not as common as infectious conjunctivitis. Allergic conjunctivitis usually causes irritation and itchiness, leading to rubbing of the eyes, even inadvertently.

Viral or Bacterial?
Viral and bacterial conjunctivitis are acute infections that can occur in your baby's eyes. Viral conjunctivitis will not respond to antibiotics, whereas bacterial infections require antibiotics. Both infections can be associated with irritation and visible inflammation of the conjunctiva. Bacterial conjunctivitis is typically associated with a colorful mucoid discharge from one or both eyes.

Drop Them In
Eyedrops may be prescribed to treat your baby's conjunctivitis. There are different kinds of eyedrops. Steroid drops will decrease inflammation, and antibiotic drops will treat a bacterial infection. To administer

eyedrops, keep your baby on her back and gently open her eyelids, placing one drop in each eye. One drop will do; that's all you need. One drop will bathe the eye with the medication.

Beyond Conjunctivitis

Most cases of conjunctivitis are mild to moderate, are not dangerous, and will resolve with time and medication (if needed). A more significant infection not to be missed is called peri-orbital cellulitis. *Peri-orbital* means "around the eye."

Cellulitis is infection of skin and soft tissue that may occur around your baby's eye and is often mistaken for conjunctivitis. Call your doctor if there is violet-red discoloration above or below her eye that is accompanied by fever.

Ear Infections

The dreaded ear infection. No doubt you have heard horror stories from friends or family members regarding ear infections. External ear infections occur in the skin of the ear canal, and they are not common in infancy. They are called otitis externa, or "swimmer's ear." The ear infections that you have heard so much about occur in the middle ear space, the space behind the ear drum, and they are called otitis media. They are not caused by wax, wind, or water in your baby's ear canal, but rather by eustachian tube dysfunction.

To explain, the eustachian tube runs from your baby's nasal passage to the middle ear space. These tubes in the face are small in size and horizontal in configuration, and their job is to move fluid back and forth between the two areas. Some babies have eustachian tubes that don't do this very well. Therefore, any congestion will cause a backup of fluid to the middle ear space, where it can sit and become infected. You can see that this is a plumbing issue! Fluid backs up, builds up, and gets infected! This is why ear infections typically follow a cold with its nasal congestion.

Congestion from food allergy or environmental allergy may also lead to a middle ear infection. Congestion from teething may lead to this as well. Any congestion can cause a buildup of fluid. Babies spend much of their time on their back, so gravity does not help to clear the fluid.

Your pediatrician may see the fluid through the eardrum, which is translucent, and the fluid may be clear or colorful when infected. The eardrum is inflamed and red, and sometimes stretched and retracted due to negative pressure. Conversely, the eardrum may be bulging outward. In either case, it is usually painful. Given enough pressure, the eardrum may open and drain the fluid. If so, you may see moist or dried discharge from the ear canal. When this occurs, pressure is actually relieved and the pain decreases dramatically.

Pressure, Pressure

If your baby ever has a middle ear infection, he will be unhappy, in large part due to pressure. The pressure behind the eardrum causes the eardrum to retract inward or to stretch outward, resulting in pain in the affected ear. This pain will cause him to feed and sleep poorly. Pain from the pressure is increased when sucking, swallowing, or lying down. On occasion, pressure will be so great as to gently perforate the eardrum, allowing fluid to drain, after which pain is relieved.

Hello in There

Your pediatrician will examine your baby's ears with an otoscope. The otoscope magnifies his view of the ear canal and the eardrum. One or both eardrums may be inflamed and red, and he may see fluid behind the translucent eardrum. He will also be able to see the anatomic landmarks of the eardrums, which may be quite distorted due to negative pressure in the eustachian tubes. Your baby's eardrum may even be blistered or perforated, with middle ear fluid draining into the ear canal.

Medication Where?

Medication should only be used if needed, as some infections are viral and won't respond to an antibiotic. Your pediatrician will know when to pre-scribe an antibiotic for your baby's middle ear infection. Oral medication is used for middle ear infections. It will travel via the bloodstream to the source of the infection. Ear drops are used to treat external canal infec-tions, or they may be recommended if an eardrum has had a perforation.

To Tube or Not To Tube

Pressure equalization (PE) tube placement may be recommended if fluid accumulation and ear infections become chronic. PE tube placement, if indicated, is performed by a surgeon and is a relatively routine procedure today. A small tube is placed in the eardrum, preventing the accumula-tion of middle ear fluid.

Tube placement and decreased fluid reduce infections and antibiotic use and help prevent expressive speech delay.

Group B Strep

One of the most serious infections in newborn babies and young infants is caused by group B streptococcus. A group B strep infection can occur in the first week of life or in infants up to three months of age. Babies are particularly at risk for this infection when their mothers are positive for group B strep. Almost half of all pregnant women carry this organism without knowledge of it or its symptoms; they are asymptomatic carriers in the vagina and cervix. That is why it is now routine to have prenatal cultures done during the last trimester of pregnancy. Group B strep can be transmitted to your baby during delivery.

Prior to delivery, pregnant women with positive cultures are given antibiotics to prevent infection in their newborn babies. If there is a history of a positive culture, the pediatrician is made aware of this when the baby is born. If a baby is infected with this organism, he can become very sick very quickly, and it is life threatening. A newborn with this infection may display signs and symptoms in the hospital nursery or once he arrives home. Early stage group B infection occurs in the first week of life. Late stage infection occurs after the first week, up to three months old. Symptoms may include irritability, lethargy, temperature instability, rapid breathing, poor feeding or vomiting, and poor sleeping. Group B strep can cause infection in the blood (bacteremia), the lungs (pneumonia), and the meninges (meningitis).

The workup required for a baby suspected of having a group B strep infection includes a chest X-ray, blood work, and a spinal tap. The baby is given intravenous antibiotics while waiting for cultures to reveal any growth. This can be life saving. The workup and admission will be done in the hospital. |167

Newborn Sepsis

If you are positive for group B strep, watch closely for signs of infection in your baby, even if antenatal antibiotics were used. In the nursery or at home in the first week of life, any significant change in your baby's behavior is important. In particular, report any changes in feeding, sleeping, and demeanor to your pediatrician right away.

Gastroenteritis

Gastroenteritis is a common infection in infants, children, and adults. *Gastro* means "stomach," *entero* means "gut," and there is that suffix *-itis* again, which means "inflamed." So gastroenteritis is inflammation of the GIT, or gastrointestinal tract. Gastroenteritis can be viral or bacterial, just like eye, ear, and throat infections. It is quite contagious via oral secretions, so your baby can catch this infection through a droplet in the air, but more often through direct contact.

As always, good hand-washing and hygiene are preventive, especially if a parent or sibling has this infection. One of many viruses is the usual culprit of a gastrointestinal infection, with incubation periods of several days to one week.

The infection can include fever, vomiting, and diarrhea, and is associated with fussiness to be certain, especially if abdominal cramps occur. Bacteria can also cause gastroenteritis, but this is less common. Your pediatrician may ask you about your water supply, or if there is any recent travel history, in particular to a foreign country.

Evaluation by your doctor is imperative with symptoms of gastroenteritis, because infants can become dehydrated rather quickly. They don't have as many fluid stores as older children or adults.

You must be prepared to recognize the signs of dehydration in your baby. The combination of fever, vomiting, and diarrhea can quickly lead to dehydration. These signs include fussiness when awake, lethargy in general, dry lips and mouth, and deceased urination. Eventually, his skin may feel doughy and not as taut.

Jelly Belly Blues

If your baby has gastroenteritis, she will be unhappy, as she may experience intermittent abdominal cramps. She may draw her legs up with the colicky, crampy pain, and she may let out gas or loosened stool. Her stool may not only be looser than usual, but it also may be watery and much more frequent. If the stool has blood or mucous in it, or if there is a large volume of it with frequent episodes, take her to your pediatrician for evaluation.

Checking In and Out

When you bring your baby to your pediatrician, he will examine her thoroughly. He will look closely for the physical findings of good hydration.

These include a moist mouth with saliva, real tears, and good skin turgor. He will palpate (push down) her abdomen to see if she is tender anywhere and to check for any mass within. If your baby has the energy to object to the exam, this is a good sign. Lethargic ill infants will not care.

Hydration

Keeping your baby well hydrated by providing fluids for her to drink can prevent the need for intravenous hydration at the hospital. Always wait at least one hour after a vomiting episode before introducing anything by mouth, as it may be rejected. In the vomiting baby, begin with small amounts given very frequently, hoping that they stay down for hydration. In the baby with diarrhea only, give large amounts of fluids infrequently, keeping up with the losses from below. An electrolyte solution may be recommended for oral rehydration. Apple juice should be avoided, as this can cause more loosened stool.

ROTAVIRUS BEWARE

There is one particular virus that can be especially dangerous and threatening to your baby. Rotavirus is a virulent organism that can cause serious infection associated with dehydration, often requiring hospitalization. Its hallmark is a large volume of frequent, foul, watery stool, which can be associated with fever. This infection can be prevented by the oral vaccine recommended for your baby in her early months.

Roseola

Roseola infantum is a common infection that can occur during your baby's first year of life. One can see this infection between six months of age and three years of age. Thankfully, this infection is not associated with disability or death. It is a harmless viral infection, and it is one that has a very typical pattern. It is contagious like any other viral infection, and it is rarely seen after age four. The typical course involves high fever for one to five days, with increases often seen in the evening. Remember that the high fever is not harmful, as it is your baby's way of fighting infection. As always, bring him to your pediatrician for evaluation.

During these days of intermittent high fevers, he may be fussy with a decreased appetite. He may also be congested, and the doctor may find that his throat is red. You may notice that your baby does not seem that ill with respect to the amount of fever. Once the fever disappears, he will immediately break out with a rash that is red and can be seen on the trunk, neck, arms, and legs. It is an impressive rash, and yet he will not seem bothered by it. The rash can last for two to seven days, and it will resolve spontaneously.

This is the typical pattern and course for the roseola infection. This infection is contagious, particularly to those his age who have not had it before, and it can be shared through secretions. Approximately 30 percent of children will get roseola before their second birthday. Those who are most at risk of catching this from your baby are his peers of the same age, six months of age up to three years of age.

The incubation period is thought to be one to two weeks, so you may alert your friends to watch their children. The infection is contagious until the rash has completely resolved in your baby.

The diagnosis is made without testing, and it is based on the history of the illness and the physical examination. The treatment of roseola is simply loving, supportive care from you. This includes fluids, dressing him lightly, and antipyretics (fever reducers) such as acetaminophen or ibuprofen to keep him comfortable.

Treat the Heat

Roseola is a viral infection associated with several days of high temperatures. High temperatures are not as significant as a rapid change in your baby's temperature. A very rapid change in temperature can induce a seizure, but this is uncommon. Avoid rapid changes in temperature by dressing your baby lightly and using antipyretic medication as needed. Remember, fever is your friend!

Rosy Roseola

Roseola is one of several viral infections that have a distinct rash associated with it. There is a distinct pattern to this illness, beginning with fevers and ending with a rash. After several days or nights of high fever, the fevers abruptly stop and the rash appears, often from head to toe. The typical rash is rosy red, flat, and blanching, and it can be dotty, spotty, and patchy. It is not usually itchy, and it is not necessary to treat the rash with any topical cream or medication.

WHAT'S IN A NAME?

Roseola is the common name for this virus, one of several infections associated with a typical rash. Roseola infantum is the widely accepted name for this infection. Exanthem subitum is the technical name for the infection. All of the names pertain to the same infection. The easiest name to remember for this infection is roseola. And remember that it ends in a rosy red rash.

Coxsackie

Coxsackie virus is another infection that can occur in your baby, and although it is uncommon, you should be aware of the signs and symptoms in case it occurs. This virus was noted long ago when it spread through a correctional facility in Coxsackie, New York. It is caused by a class of viruses known as enteroviruses, which are found in the digestive tract. It is quite contagious, especially from unwashed hands or anything contaminated by feces.

The usual time for this virus to flourish and cause infection is during the summer and early fall, but it can occur at any time of year. Outbreaks can occur in day care facilities or in preschool settings, and it may spread rapidly among peers. The infection can be spread by shared secretions, which can be transmitted directly from coughing, drooling, shared toys, and so on. Good hand-washing is imperative.

The incubation period is probably three days to one week, and then the fun begins. Your baby may become fussy and warm to touch due to fever as she fights the infection. Appetite is always decreased due to sores in the mouth or throat, which are painful. Your pediatrician may detect several small sores in the mouth or throat that appear red, blistery, and angry. This is called herpangina. The sores are typically found on the palate and in the

HAND, FOOT, AND MOUTH

Hand, foot, and mouth disease is the name for the Coxsackie virus when it causes blisters on the hands and feet. This is not to be confused with hoof and mouth disease. Although hoof and mouth disease is also caused by a virus, this infection affects only mammals with cloven hooves! Animals spread hoof and mouth disease to each other much as children spread the coxsackie virus to each other, but the two infections are totally unrelated.

tonsillar area. Small blisters on the hands and feet can occur, and they are sometimes painful to touch. When blisters occur on the hands and feet, the child has what is called hand, foot, and mouth disease.

Spot the Difference

The spots or sores in the mouth from Coxsackie viral infections are typical and rarely misdiagnosed. The spots on the skin may be confused with insect bites, pustulosis, or other viral infections such as chicken pox. Coxsackie infection causes small blisters (vesicles) that appear to be under the skin. They have a pink or red halo. These spots can be seen on the palms of her hands, between fingers, on the soles of her feet, and between the toes.

Spot-On Treatment

Coxsackie infection will resolve without treatment, but you can help your baby to be comfortable. Keep her dressed lightly and cool, and keep her well hydrated with fluids; her appetite for solids will return later. Avoid spicy or acidic foods, as these may cause discomfort in her mouth. Cold food items can be soothing. Analgesics (pain relievers) will be helpful and should be used as needed. Wash your hands well, especially after changing her diaper.

Pneumonia

Pneumonia is an infection that occurs in the lungs, and although it is not common in infancy, it is very dangerous when it does occur. When your baby has a cold, it usually resolves without any complication. Pneumonia can follow an upper respiratory infection, or cold, because mucoid secretions are a terrific breeding ground for bacteria. They can multiply and cause a localized infection in one of the lobes of the lung.

Pneumonia can be caused by a virus or a bacteria, and one of the most commonly implicated bacteria is pneumococcal strep. This is a very aggressive organism that can cause a kind of pneumonia associated with great disability and that can cause life-threatening infection. It is not uncommon for this organism to cause an empyema, a collection of pus in the lungs that must be drained surgically. Thankfully, your baby will receive four vaccinations in his first year of life to protect him against this form of streptococcus. Pneumonia can cause your baby to become ill quickly, so be on the lookout for certain signs and symptoms.

This kind of infection usually follows a cold and congestion, but it does not have to. It may also be associated with conjunctivitis (pink eye) or otitis (ear infection), but it may not. The hallmark is a cough that becomes more and more frequent and will progress to occur both day and night. It may be dry, harsh, or moist in quality. The quality of the cough can reflect the kind of pneumonia that is present. Suffice it to say that any coughing infant must be examined by the pediatrician.

As with other significant infections, your baby with pneumonia will be clingy, fussy, and febrile. Fever is almost always present as he tries to fight the infection. His breathing will be rapid, and his cough will be persistent. Appetite is decreased, activity is low, and sleep is disrupted. The increased work of breathing leads to all of these compromises to his usual routine. If any of these symptoms are present, bring your baby to his pediatrician for evaluation as soon as possible.

Chlamydia Pneumonia

Chlamydia trachomatis is another bacteria that can cause pneumonia in young infants. This organism is sexually transmitted, and it causes infection in hosts of all ages. When infants get pneumonia from this organism, it has been inadvertently spread to them from their mother. Chlamydial pneumonia is often associated with conjunctivitis, and both are treated with antibiotics.

Viral Pneumonia

Bacteria are not the only cause of pneumonia; viruses can cause pneumonia with the same or similar symptoms. Adenovirus, influenza virus, and parainfluenza virus can all cause pneumonia in your baby. RSV, or respiratory syncytial virus, can cause a pneumonitis called bronchiolitis. Although antibiotics don't treat viruses, initial treatment will include empiric antibiotics to ensure your baby's safety from bacteria.

Bugs and Drugs

If pneumonia is suspected, your baby will be evaluated by a workup that includes a chest X-ray and blood work. Hospitalization is usually required for IV hydration, IV antibiotics, and supplemental oxygen if needed. Depending on the age of the baby at the time of diagnosis, different viruses or bacteria may be the culprit. In order to cover all of the possible offending (and offensive) organisms, broad-spectrum antibiotics are used.

Meningitis

Meningitis is a word that brings fear to most parents who hear it. You may have heard that it is a possible cause of fever, headache, vomiting, and a stiff neck. Your baby may have some of these symptoms, but she cannot tell you with words, so we must be prepared to identify this serious infection.

The meninges are the covering of the brain and spinal cord, and as you know, the suffix *-itis* means "inflamed"—hence the term *meningitis*. A virus or bacteria can cause this inflammation and infection, and it must be treated quickly and aggressively. A viral meningitis is not as dangerous as a bacterial meningitis, unless it occurs in the early months of life when your baby's immune system is not as strong. These organisms may exist in the mouths of otherwise healthy infants and children, but they go on to cause infection when they seed the bloodstream and affect the body more deeply.

Babies with a meningeal infection will be irritable and inconsolable. They will have temperature instability (hot or cold), and they will feed poorly. Their skin may have a mottled appearance if they are not having normal blood flow with their circulation. This is a sign of significant infection. If your baby is displaying any signs or symptoms of meningitis, bring her to your pediatrician right away. Your doctor will examine her thoroughly, and if meningitis is suspected, he will order immediate testing.

The infant with meningitis may display signs of increased intracerebral pressure. When pressure rises in the brain, she will have headaches and therefore seem to be in pain, and she may vomit. Her anterior fontanel (soft spot) may be full or bulging. The fontanel may normally be full when she is supine, but fullness when she is upright, combined with other symptoms, is of great concern.

If your baby is ill and her pediatrician suspects significant infection, a thorough workup will follow. If meningitis is suspected, the evaluation will include a lumbar puncture, or spinal tap. Please don't be afraid of these words, and don't hesitate to allow a spinal tap to be done to your baby. It is a must. The tiny needle is placed in a safe place to withdraw fluid without any damage to the spinal cord. When a sick baby or child is evaluated for serious infection, body fluids are obtained and sent for culture. Laboratories can culture fluids to grow viral and bacterial organisms, which will then help direct the treatment. Culture results usually take several days to return after growing an organism from either blood or spinal fluid. If a bacterial organism is identified, a sensitivity evaluation is provided so that the doctor may confirm the correct antibiotic to use.

Once the final spinal fluid culture result is received, treatment can be streamlined for the baby with meningitis. Viral meningitis does not require an antibiotic, so the medication may be discontinued. Bacterial meningitis must be fully treated with the appropriate antibiotic based on the culture and sensitivity. The duration of antibiotic therapy in the hospital and at home will be determined and advised.

CHAPTER FOURTEEN

Developmental Issues and Specialist Consultations

There are few things in life more thrilling and fulfilling than watching your children grow, develop, change, and thrive. You will be in awe as each developmental milestone is reached, particularly during his first year of life. Of course, when we speak of development, it is wise to remember that your baby's development really begins with conception. The development of the nervous system begins with the neural tube during the first month of embryonic life. As the fetus grows, the brain and all of the fetus's organs are formed by the end of third trimester. Maintaining a good state of health during your pregnancy is imperative to ensuring your baby's intrauterine health and safety. Any significant medical issues that you may have can affect him and his future. Work closely with your obstetrician as always.

Once you have delivered your baby, you will be monitoring his ongoing development with your pediatrician. This will include his physical, social, emotional, language, and intellectual development. Along with your partner and other loved ones, you and the doctor will be the primary team to observe this development over time. Medical issues may alter normal development, and these have to be considered as your baby is observed. For example, prematurity or any perinatal difficulties can affect development. Also, heredity may play a role in development as certain traits can be passed along genetically. Along with these factors, development is dependent in large part on relationships, in particular your baby's relationship with you. Your interactions will always be very important in his ongoing development, especially in the first year of life. Also, the environment that you and his caretakers provide will greatly affect his development as you interact each day. Normal development will be most encouraged as you provide a safe, loving, nurturing, and stimulating environment in your home.

Home on the Range

When you are watching your child's development, please remember that she is a unique individual, different from every other. Her development may vary greatly from what you recall in one or more of her siblings. It may also vary greatly compared to the development of her peers. Some babies are ahead and some are behind the average. Those who are ahead are not better. The most important thing to remember is that there is a range of normal for each and every milestone that is attained. The range of normal for any milestone has been determined by years of study in the field of child development. If your pediatrician assures you that your baby is within the normal range in all of the areas of her development, then rest in comfort.

Today more than at any other time, pediatricians are devoted to noting any delays in development, because they know that early intervention is the best intervention. Your pediatrician will be monitoring your baby's development in several ways. First, he will be asking you questions about what the baby has been doing since the previous well-child visit. He will also be watching closely during each visit, before and after the examination. The evaluation really begins as he enters the room and first sees your baby in your arms. As the visit is being summarized, he will let you know if there are any developmental concerns. There may be no issue, or something to watch closely, or an issue to address with an evaluation. Trust your instincts as well. Pediatricians want to hear your concerns, because you know your baby better than anyone else. If you feel that something is not right, please speak up. Just remember that your baby is fine if she is "home on the range." Please refer to the following normal ranges for achieving developmental milestones.

Motor Range

There is a normal range for each motor milestone that your baby attains, whether it is gross motor or fine motor. Some babies roll over at four months, most roll over at six months, and some roll over at eight months of age. Your baby may crawl between six and nine months, but some skip crawling and pull to stand without having crawled at all. Most babies take first steps around thirteen months old, but the range can be nine to sixteen months of age.

Speech Range

Another range of normal to consider is in the area of speech and language; it is rare for receptive speech (what your baby hears and processes) to be delayed. Expressive speech begins with the newborn cry and follows with delightful oohs, coos, and goos. Babble leads to happy screeching, followed by monosyllables such as da, ba, and ma, usually by nine months of age. Most babies use these syllables in context between twelve and fifteen months, but some do so earlier.

Social Range

Social interaction has a range of normal as well. Most babies will attain the responsive social smile by two months of age. Your baby will probably be chuckling with mild laughter at four months old, but many will do this at six months old. Some babies begin to wave hello or good-bye at nine months, whereas most will do so by their first birthday. If your baby reads social cues progressively during her first year, she is developing well. Don't rely on exact timing for each milestone to be attained.

Intellectual Range

Almost all babies have normal reflex actions such as sucking with their mouths and grasping with their hands in the first weeks of life. As they grow, infants will notice more and respond more to their environment with each passing day, week, and month. There is also a range of normal for cognitive development. Babies may differ in their recognition and grasp of concepts. Object permanence, or the understanding of the existence of things they don't see, can also vary from baby to baby.

Medical Impact

Developmental delays are not common. Studies in the field of child development have determined the average age of attainment for every milestone, with an acceptable range of normal for each. According to these studies, approximately 3 to 5 percent of babies will not attain a milestone at the average time, but only a small percentage of these babies actually have abnormal development. Those that do may have a medical reason. When a delay in any area of development is evident, your pediatrician will seek a reason to explain it. The treatment, or intervention, for that delay may not change based upon a diagnosis, but a cause will be sought for a better understanding. For example, prior to newborn screening, congenital hypothyroidism (underactive thyroid gland function) led to impaired intellectual development. Hypothyroidism was formerly an unknown factor in a baby's development, and such impairment should no longer occur. Other medical issues are known, and they can have a significant impact on development.

Prematurity predisposes a baby to developmental delay in all areas, depending on the gestational age of the baby at birth, and also depending on the baby's hospital course after birth. For example, if a preterm baby has a complication such as intraventricular hemorrhage (bleeding in the brain), he is at risk for developmental delay. However, it is amazing not only how many preterm infants survive, but also how many live their lives without complications or subsequent delays thanks to advances in neonatal medicine. In fact, a preterm baby with an uncomplicated course may only have relative motor delay due to his physical size. Time alone compensates for this delay, as the baby will eventually catch up in his physical growth. In rare instances, perinatal asphyxia (lack of oxygen around the time of birth) occurs, which can have a great impact on future development. Thankfully, this is uncommon today due to good obstetrical and neonatal care.

Hypoxia

Hypoxia is lack of oxygen, an uncommon occurrence in both preterm babies and full-term babies. The brain does not receive enough oxygen when perinatal asphyxia and hypoxia occur. When a baby is hypoxic for a long enough period of time, brain function is compromised due to the lack of adequate oxygen. Developmental delay is highly associated with a history of a hypoxic event.

Consultation

If you or your pediatrician suspect a delay in development, a consultation with a subspecialist may be recommended. Pediatric developmentalists are pediatricians who have undergone training to be subspecialists in child development. Pediatric neurologists are neurologists who have undergone training to become subspecialists in pediatric brain function. Any baby with a developmental delay deserves an evaluation by one or both of these subspecialists.

Specific Delays

During your baby's first year of life and beyond, you and your pediatrician will be watching your baby's developmental progress very closely. You will be pleased if she is within the normal range of development as she achieves each milestone. She may have a delay in a certain area of development. One of the most common delays that parents and pediatricians encounter is a delay in expressive speech. Remember that each baby differs and develops at her own rate. Expressive speech pertains to how babies communicate. As your baby grows and communicates, she will go from cooing, to babbling, to monosyllables, to words in context by fifteen to eighteen months. If this progress is delayed, she deserves an evaluation.

Barring a medical issue, an expressive speech delay may have no known cause, or it may be that this baby is your second or third child and everyone around her is doing the speaking for her! Gross motor delays are also not infrequent. Your baby may not pull to stand at nine months, and she may not cruise, stand alone, and walk at thirteen months. Some babies begin to toddle between fifteen and eighteen months. If her gross motor development is lagging, your doctor may recommend an evaluation, and the cause may be hypotonia, or low muscle tone. Low tone may also affect her ability to eat and swallow. This is known as oromotor hypotonia, and it can affect speech development as well.

Global developmental delay can occur as a result of any compromise to the central nervous system. Global delay involves every area of development, and it is usually associated with lower intellectual function. The achievement of all milestones will be delayed. There are many causes of global developmental delay. They may be genetic or related to perinatal events.

Talking Woman

Speech development is a joy to watch and to hear, and expressive speech delay is quite common. Don't panic if your baby is delayed compared to siblings or friends. They may be speaking for her. If she has normal receptive speech and language development, the expressive speech usually follows with time. Isolated expressive speech and language delay is quite remedial with therapy provided by a qualified speech therapist.

Walking Man

Your baby will probably let go of you and walk between twelve and fifteen months of age. He will generally be trying to climb stairs and anything else in sight at that fun and adventurous age. If he is lagging in the gross motor or fine motor areas, he should be evaluated to see if he has low muscle tone. Physical therapists address gross motor delays, and occupational therapists address fine motor delays.

Oromotor Hypotonia

Low muscle tone can affect any muscle in the body, including the muscles in your baby's mouth. Beginning in early infancy, oromotor tone is very important for the control of secretions as your baby sucks and swallows. Low oromotor tone can account for excessive drooling, poor feeding, poor weight gain, and speech delay. Oromotor hypotonia is addressed with many techniques utilized by speech therapists who specialize in this area.

Global Delay

Global developmental delay is uncommon, but it is a very serious developmental concern. All areas of development are affected, with delays in speech, motor, social, and intellectual development. Pediatricians will fully evaluate any baby suspected of having global developmental delay. Evaluation consists of lab studies, imaging (such as MRIs), and subspecialty consultations. Known causes of global developmental delay include serious infection, genetic syndromes, metabolic disorders, and prematurity with a complicated course.

Autism

Autism is a highly charged word today, and that is because it is such a devastating diagnosis to hear or to have, and because of the controversy that continues regarding its origin. Autism, now referred to as autism spectrum disorder, is a diagnosis given to a child who has displayed a variety of features inconsistent with normal development. It is now considered to be a spectrum, with individuals differing in their particular features and their severity. Most experts agree that all children affected by autism are impaired in their ability to communicate and that they have difficulty connecting socially.

Children with classic autism have delayed speech and may remain nonverbal. They may have motor delay as well. They will usually have poor eye contact with others, even family members, and they may have repetitive mannerisms such as frequent hand-flapping. Autistic children will often concentrate on a particular area of interest to the point of obsession. High-functioning individuals have normal or even higher-than-normal intellect. Remember that this is a spectrum disorder. Delays in a baby's or a child's developmental milestones in association with any concerns regarding socialization and/or cognitive development should prompt evaluation.

The cause of autism remains unknown. It is still thought to be largely idiopathic, even after years of dedicated research and study by experts. Others have postulated that environmental factors may play a role in the development of autism, but research has found no significant connection. Vaccines and an individual's unique reaction to them and to preservatives formerly used in vaccine production have been questioned, but still no real connection has been found. Many therapies that are considered to be experimental have been utilized in children with autism with the hope of recovery or cure, but none have been proven to achieve this result. The goal of therapy should always be directed to the individual needs of each autistic child, with any and all safe, accepted therapies offered.

What's in a Name?

The word *autistic* has long been used to describe an individual who has impaired social skills and communication. Today we use ASD, or autism spectrum disorder, to describe autism, because there is a spectrum of features that one can display. As with any area of development, an individual may be affected to a mild, moderate, or severe degree. When ASD is suspected, subspecialty consultations will help to diagnose accurately, and services are provided.

PDD/NOS

Pervasive Developmental Disorder/Not Otherwise Specified (PDD/NOS) describes a child who has some but not all of the features of classic autism. Usually diagnosed by the age of four, this is considered to be on the mild side of the spectrum.

With PDD/NOS, a child may have poor social interaction and repetitive behaviors, and he may be overly sensitive to his surroundings. Therapy for children with PDD/NOS is individualized and can include behavioral therapy, medication, and social skills training.

Asperger's Syndrome

Named after an Austrian pediatrician, Asperger's syndrome is thought to be a form of "high-functioning autism." Children with Asperger's syndrome usually do not have delayed milestones, and they are of normal if not superior intellect. As with others on the autistic spectrum, these children have difficulty reading social cues, leading to difficulty with social interaction. Treatment is again individualized and can include social skills training and behavioral therapy.

Autism Treatment

Every child is a unique individual with different needs, strengths, and weaknesses, and treatment must be individualized. ABA (applied behavior analysis) is commonly used. ABA devotes several hours per day to analysis at home or at a center. The objective of ABA is to engage in repetitive actions and behaviors in a given environment with a reward system for reinforcement. In addition to ABA, services by speech therapists, physical therapists, occupational therapists, and special educators are used as needed.

Early Intervention

If you or your pediatrician have any concerns about the developmental progress of your little one, the concerns should be addressed sooner rather than later. As noted earlier, you may be worried about one or more areas of your baby's development, and her doctor may reassure you that all is well, with the understanding that you and he will continue to monitor together. As time passes, and if you remain concerned, the issue will be readdressed. Mothers know their babies; you will not be ignored. If your pediatrician has a concern about development, he will bring it up at the well visit. If you were not already aware of the issue, he will fully apprise you and do one of two things. He may wish to watch closely until the next well visit to see if the concern remains, or he may recommend a consultation with a subspecialist. If a subspecialty consultation is not needed, he may recommend an early intervention evaluation.

Early Intervention (EI) is a voluntary program offered in every state to any eligible child between birth and three years of age. It is available through your state or county health department. When either a parent or pediatrician has a developmental concern, the parent simply contacts the health department, and the process begins. An ongoing service provider will be assigned to oversee this process for you and your baby. Evaluations ensue depending on the area of concern. The evaluations may take place in your home or at an evaluation center. The personnel performing the evaluations with you and your baby are professionals in their fields. Again, depending on the issue, they may be speech therapists, occupational therapists, physical therapists, social workers, psychologists, or special educators. After the evaluation process has been completed, a meeting will take place to discuss the results.

The Meeting

Once your baby's evaluations have been completed, a meeting will take place in order to review all of the results. An Early Intervention specialist from the state or county will be present, along with your ongoing service coordinator. In addition, one or more of the evaluators will be present in case there are any questions about their evaluations. You may have your baby with you at this meeting, but she is not required to be there.

Who Is Eligible?

Eligibility for services depends on the results of the evaluations. Your baby may not qualify for subsidized services. Qualification for subsidized services is based on your state or county's specific regulations. Your baby may be in need of a specific service, but the cost of that service may not be covered by the government. According to your state's regulations, babies must be deficient in more than one domain in order to qualify.

Taxing and Taxing

It is of course a very good thing if your baby does not qualify for services after an EI evaluation. You may feel slighted since you have a concern and you pay taxes to support these programs. However, the Early Intervention program was designed to give services to those infants and children with the most significant special needs. If your baby does have a need for a certain therapy but does not qualify under EI regulations, she may receive that therapy privately.

Automatic or Not

Some babies are automatically eligible for Early Intervention services, although all must go through the evaluation process. Babies who are born prematurely and are under a certain birth weight (per your state) are automatically eligible.

Babies with certain syndromes are automatically eligible for services—for example, those with trisomy 21, or Down syndrome. Babies considered medically fragile, such as those with spina bifida, may be automatically eligible.

When Do You Need a Specialist?

Names may change, but the system remains the same. Your pediatrician is a specialist in the field of general pediatrics, trained to specialize in the medical care of newborn infants to young adults. If a pediatrician wishes to subspecialize, he may do so with additional training in the pediatric subspecialty of his choice. There are many pediatric subspecialties, just as there are many subspecialties in adult medicine. It is a blessing for general pediatricians and their patients to have subspecialists available to address specific needs. The pediatric subspecialists are consultants, and they have special interest and expertise in one certain area of pediatric medicine. In today's medical milieu, you may hear different titles in the name game, so be prepared and try not to be confused. Your general pediatrician may be called a PCP, or primary care provider, and the subspecialist you may be consulting might be called a specialist. Don't be concerned with the titles, as the roles they play in your baby's life are as we have described them. Pediatric subspecialists may or may not be located in your community, but they are certain to be found in association with any medical school or large tertiary care medical center.

Pediatric subspecialists are available to us in medical areas and surgical areas. Many will divide their time between clinical medicine and academic medicine, particularly if they work in association with a school of medicine. Clinical medicine involves seeing patients in their office when consulted by your general pediatrician, and making recommendations to families with regard to the issue at hand. Academic medicine refers to the teaching of medical students, interns, and residents and active involvement in medical research.

In addition to pediatric medical and surgical subspecialties, there are mental health professionals who may specialize in the care of children. Social workers have master's degrees, and they are trained to evaluate children and provide counseling for them. Psychologists have doctorate degrees, and after completing their general psychology education, they may specialize in child and adolescent psychology. Psychiatrists have medical degrees and are trained in general psychiatry, and they may then specialize in child and adolescent psychiatry.

PEDIATRIC MEDICAL SUBSPECIALTIES

* Adolescent Health
* Allergy/Immunology
* Critical Care
* Dentistry
* Dermatology
* Development
* Emergency Medicine
* Endocrinology
* Gastroenterology
* Genetics

* Hematology/Oncology
* Hospital Medicine
* Infectious Disease
* Neonatology
* Nephrology
* Neurology
* Pulmonology
* Radiology
* Rheumatology
* Sports Medicine

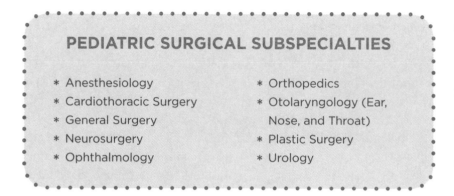

PEDIATRIC SURGICAL SUBSPECIALTIES

* Anesthesiology
* Cardiothoracic Surgery
* General Surgery
* Neurosurgery
* Ophthalmology

* Orthopedics
* Otolaryngology (Ear, Nose, and Throat)
* Plastic Surgery
* Urology

Neonatology

If pediatric consultants are recommended, there are many available to assist you and your pediatrician in the care of your baby. We will review the most common ones that you may be referred to in your baby's first year of life. Beginning with the newborn period, the neonatologist may be needed if your baby is premature or ill in any way following your delivery. The neonatologist is in the hospital and available for consultation, and if necessary she can admit your baby to the neonatal intensive care unit (NICU) for close monitoring and specialized care by highly trained neonatal nursing staff.

The neonatologist is a physician who has completed post-graduate training in general pediatrics and a fellowship in neonatal medicine. Her subspecialty concentrates on newborn infants, especially those who are premature or critically ill. The neonatologist works with the obstetrician if there are concerns about an expected baby prior to a delivery. Neonatologists are trained to evaluate and care for babies with the most complex neonatal issues in the intensive care unit setting.

Critical Care

In rare instances, babies may become significantly ill during their first year. If your baby does become significantly ill, he may need to be admitted to a pediatric intensive care unit (PICU). The consultant in the PICU is a subspecialist in pediatric critical care. This subspecialist is an intensivist in charge of caring for infants through young adults in the pediatric intensive care unit. An intensivist is a physician with special training in the care of patients who require an intensive care setting due to a high level of acute illness. The pediatric intensivist oversees the monitoring of critically ill infants and children by the critical care nursing staff to ensure the highest level of care.

This subspecialist is first trained in general pediatrics and then completes a fellowship in pediatric critical care. He focuses on the critically ill pediatric patient from infancy through adolescence. Like the neonatologist, this physician is highly skilled at handling life-threatening situations for children. He directs and coordinates the care of patients who require treatment and monitoring in the pediatric intensive care unit setting.

Hospitalist

If your baby needs to be admitted to the hospital but is not critically ill, he will be admitted to the pediatric ward and cared for by a pediatric hospitalist. This subspecialist has chosen to subspecialize in pediatric hospital medicine. In contrast to the general pediatrician, the pediatric hospitalist is in charge of any infant, child, or young adult admitted to the ward. She works with specialized pediatric nursing staff, and together they offer complete care to sick pediatric patients of all ages. Your pediatrician may admit and care for her patients on a pediatric ward herself, and she is well equipped to do so, but many hospitals now have a pediatric hospitalist program in place, offering constant in-house availability and attention.

The hospitalist is a physician who has been trained in general pediatrics and who chooses to practice hospital-based medicine. She is highly qualified to care for pediatric patients of all ages who require hospitalization in the general pediatric ward. The pediatric hospitalist monitors admitted patients closely, and she can stabilize patients who need to be transferred to a critical care setting.

The hospitalist oversees the care of hospitalized children, working with nursing staff, respiratory therapists, surgeons, and other subspecialists.

WHEN DO WE NEED THEM?

Neonatologist: prematurity, respiratory distress syndrome, infection, genetic syndromes, congenital malformations, and high-risk deliveries

Critical Care: overwhelming infection, significant injuries, post-operative care, diabetic ketoacidosis, status asthmaticus, and near drowning

Hospitalist: gastroenteritis/dehydration, asthma exacerbation, bronchiolitis, infection, post-operative care, pneumonia, and hyperbilirubinemia

Each of these highly trained subspecialists works with families and their pediatricians to ensure good communication and consistency of care.

Emergency Medicine

When a baby or child presents to the emergency department, she is cared for by a physician and his team trained in emergency medicine. Teaching hospitals and large community hospitals may have pediatric emergency physicians available. They are pediatricians whose subspecialty is devoted to the care of acutely ill or injured infants, children, and adolescents. They are experts in the stabilization and treatment of seriously ill patients in potentially life-threatening circumstances.

A pediatric emergency physician first trains in general pediatrics and then completes a fellowship in pediatric emergency medicine. He is highly skilled in life-saving procedures for acutely ill or injured pediatric patients of all ages. This physician and his team stabilize and treat patients, resulting in either discharge home, or admission to the pediatric ward or the intensive care unit. Emergency physicians work with families to inform, educate, and comfort them during emergency situations involving their children.

Surgery

The pediatric surgeon may be consulted whenever a baby or child has a need for evaluation and care that is of a surgical nature. These surgeons perform procedures on preterm or full-term infants with hernias, older infants with intestinal blockage, and older children with appendicitis, to name just a few diagnoses. They can repair seen and unseen congenital malformations in babies. Pediatric surgeons operate in community hospitals and in large tertiary care centers.

The pediatric surgeon is a physician trained in general surgery who then chooses to complete additional training in pediatric surgery. Pediatric surgeons are trained to perform surgical procedures on preterm and full-term infants, children, and adolescents. Depending on the procedure and the patient, they can perform surgery with minimally invasive or invasive techniques. These surgeons work closely with pediatricians, hospitalists, and intensivists to achieve coordinated care for pediatric patients.

Urology

Pediatric urologists are surgeons who specialize in genito-urinary issues in babies and children. They will be consulted to evaluate genital abnormalities such as penile malformations and undescended testicles. These urologists will also be consulted to evaluate babies who have a prenatal diagnosis of a kidney malformation.

Pediatric urologists are surgeons trained in urology who then train specifically in pediatric genito-urinary surgery. They may be consulted in the nursery prior to circumcision if your baby boy's penis or foreskin is malformed in any way. Prenatal diagnosis of a kidney malformation on ultrasound will prompt consultation after delivery if the issue persists. Pediatric urologists evaluate babies with common and uncommon diagnoses, such as undescended testes and ambiguous genitalia.

Ear, Nose, and Throat

Pediatric ear, nose, and throat (ENT) physicians are surgeons who may be consulted for any issue involving these areas of your baby's body. They are otolaryngologists who operate on infants and children. They may be consulted to evaluate babies with congenital malformations, upper airway obstruction, and the very common chronic middle ear fluid and infection. Known as pediatric ENT specialists, they have subspecialized in the ENT care of children. All of these surgeons can be trusted to give the highest level of care to your baby or child, working closely with your pediatrician.

They explain the need for procedures and any risks involved so that all of your questions are answered thoroughly.

A pediatric otolaryngologist, or ear, nose, and throat surgeon, has completed subspecialty training to care for pediatric patients. This is the surgeon who performs tube placement in the infant or child with chronic middle ear fluid. She is also the surgeon who will perform adenoidectomy and/or tonsillectomy in children with upper airway obstruction. These surgeons work with pediatric anesthesiologists to ensure the safest care for your baby in the operating room.

Development

If your baby has a significant developmental concern, your pediatrician will probably recommend a consultation with a subspecialist. You may be referred to a pediatric developmentalist for consultation. She can assess your baby's developmental progress as it compares to normal ranges of development in all areas, and she can further recommend any necessary services that are available for infants and children with special needs.

The pediatric developmentalist first trains as a general pediatrician and then completes a fellowship to subspecialize in child development. She is the subspecialist who assesses the overall development of infants and children. Skilled in assessment of needs, she may recommend certain therapies or evaluations by other experts in related service areas. Developmentalists are also experts who can be consulted when older children have issues related to attention and learning.

Neurology

If your pediatrician has a concern with regard to your baby's neurologic status, she will refer you to a pediatric neurologist. This subspecialist will be consulted for issues such as seizures in infants and children, and he can also comment on development since many developmental issues are neurologically related. For example, babies with very low muscle tone will be referred for evaluation because this issue impacts their overall development. Pediatric neurologists are also experts in issues that arise in older children, such as migraine disorders and all forms of epilepsy.

The child neurologist is first trained as a general neurologist and then chooses to have additional fellowship training for infants and children. This subspecialist should be consulted if you and your pediatrician have any concerns about your baby's neurologic (brain) function. Rare issues such as perinatal asphyxia, brain hemorrhage in preterm infants, and seizures all prompt consultation with the neurologist.

Neurosurgery

Pediatric neurosurgeons may be consulted during the early months of your baby's infancy if the baby's skull size and shape are of concern to you or your doctor. Plagiocephaly is a term describing asymmetrical skull development, which may prompt consultation if the condition is significant. It is usually caused by a favoring of position, leading to unevenness of the skull since the bones of the skull have not yet fused. The neurosurgeon can differentiate this positional molding from craniosynostosis, a rare occurrence of premature closure of the cranial suture lines.

A pediatric neurosurgeon first trains as a general surgeon, then as a neurosurgeon, and then subspecializes in neurosurgery for infants and children. Pediatric neurosurgeons may be found in association with medical schools and large tertiary care centers. They will be consulted for plagiocephaly, trauma, tumor, spinal deformities, and craniosynostosis. On occasion, a baby with positional molding, or plagiocephaly, will be advised to wear a helmet to reshape her head.

Genetics

Genetics is an important subspecialty of pediatrics, although the need for consultation is rare. The geneticist will be consulted when there is evidence on a baby's physical examination that is suggestive of a particular genetic syndrome. Geneticists are skilled in the evaluation of patients who may have a chromosomal abnormality, and they can advise parents and pediatricians regarding the appropriate multidisciplinary care that is often necessary.

A subspecialist in genetics first trains in general pediatrics and then subspecializes in the field of genetics. She is an expert in the field of genetics and heredity, to which many syndromes in children can be traced. The geneticist will be consulted in the rare instance of a baby born with abnormalities of his structure, chemistry, or brain development. The genetics expert is highly skilled to work with families of children with special needs who require specific genetic counseling.

197

Cardiology

One of the most commonly consulted subspecialists in pediatric medicine is the pediatric cardiologist. Heart murmurs are quite common in infancy and childhood, and they are usually benign, innocent flow murmurs, but pediatricians are always careful to confirm this with a consultation. Thankfully, significant congenital cardiac anomalies are uncommon. Cardiologists are experts in cardiac function. They evaluate fetal hearts with ultrasound, and they see older children with rhythm disturbances as well.

The pediatric cardiologist is first trained as a general pediatrician and then completes a fellowship in pediatric cardiology. Pediatric cardiologists are experts in all aspects of cardiac function in premature infants, full-term infants, children, adolescents, and young adults. If your baby has a heart murmur, this subspecialist may be consulted, and his evaluation may include a chest X-ray, a cardiogram, and an echocardiogram. Although complex congenital heart malformations are rare occurrences, the pediatric cardiologist is the one to make the diagnosis and direct the care.

Gastroenterology

Pediatric gastroenterologists subspecialize in gastrointestinal function and nutrition, and they may be consulted if your baby has significant spitting or reflux, colic, constipation, or failure to thrive. These entities and abdominal pain in older children can be frustrating for patients and their parents, and may warrant a consultation. Intestinal obstruction is rare.

The pediatric gastroenterologist first trains as a general pediatrician and then completes a fellowship in pediatric gastroenterology. He has expertise in nutrition, liver issues, and all matters pertaining to the digestive system in infants, children, and adolescents. He may be consulted for babies with reflux, significant constipation in infants or children, and food allergy issues. Less-common reasons for a consultation with a pediatric gastroenterologist include chronic diarrhea, failure to thrive, malabsorption, lactose intolerance, and liver disease.

Pulmonology

The pediatric pulmonologist is another subspecialist available to evaluate babies with both common and uncommon diagnoses. Pediatric pulmonologists are experts in lung function and can render opinions and recommendations regarding the wheezing infant or child as well as asthmatic older children. They will be consulted in rare situations, such as when babies experience broncho-pulmonary dysplasia following prematurity with a complicated course, or when a child has cystic fibrosis.

This subspecialist also completes the three-year general pediatric residency and then chooses to do a fellowship in pediatric pulmonary medicine. The pediatric pulmonologist can be consulted for any concern that pertains to your baby's breathing, lung function, or any uncommon lung disease. Common consultations may be made for recurrent wheezing in infancy, apnea, and chronic cough and asthma in older children. The pediatric pulmonologist will diagnose and treat babies with chronic lung issues resulting from prematurity, recurrent pneumonia, and cystic fibrosis.

Radiology

Radiologists are specialists in radiology who train to have expertise in obtaining and interpreting many imaging modalities, including X-rays, CT scans, ultrasounds, and MRIs. Imaging techniques and studies differ for infants and children because your little ones are not simply small adults. This is why radiologists can subspecialize in pediatric radiology.

The pediatric radiologist first completes training in diagnostic radiology and then chooses to complete additional training in pediatric radiology. She is then an expert in the use of today's available imaging for children, including X-rays, ultrasounds, CT scans, and MRIs. The pediatric radiologist will recommend the right imaging for your little patient, ensure its safety, and make an accurate diagnosis.

Pediatric radiologists are experts in both adult and pediatric radiology, and they may be found at large children's hospitals and tertiary care centers.

Dermatology

The pediatric dermatologist is a dermatologist with a special interest in the skin disorders of childhood. Pediatric dermatologists have special expertise in the diagnosis and treatment of all skin conditions from infancy to young adulthood. The general dermatologists in your community may be consulted, as they probably see both pediatric and adult patients. They may be consulted to evaluate congenital birthmarks or infantile eczema that is out of control.

The pediatric dermatologist first trains in general dermatology and then completes one or more years of fellowship in pediatric dermatology. You may not have this subspecialist in your community, and most general dermatologists are comfortable treating children. Pediatric dermatologists can be found in urban settings, at major medical centers, in association with medical schools, and at children's hospitals. Today, dermatologists are trained to diagnose and treat skin conditions with medication, cryotherapy, excision and biopsy, and laser therapy.

Ophthalmology

Pediatric ophthalmologists subspecialize in your baby's eyes and their function. From congenital issues such as ptosis (lid lag) and dacryostenosis (blocked tear duct), to vision correction in children, to rare occurrences such as cataracts and tumors, the pediatric ophthalmologist is the subspecialist to be called.

The pediatric ophthalmologist first trains in ophthalmology and then chooses to complete a one-year fellowship in pediatric ophthalmology. Your pediatrician will call on this physician to evaluate any possible eye disorder, congenital or otherwise. She may be consulted if your baby is born with ptosis or dacryostenosis, or if your baby should suffer any eye injury. She will diagnose and treat vision disturbance and can surgically treat issues involving muscle weakness.

Orthopedics

The pediatric orthopedist may be consulted if your baby has a congenital hip dislocation or if there is an uncommon deformity such as club feet. Of course, he is also available to evaluate intoeing or outtoeing, significant tibial torsion (bowing of the lower legs), and any fracture that may occur as your baby grows.

Pediatric orthopedists are first trained in general orthopedic surgery, followed by subspecialty training in pediatric bone disease and disorders in all pediatric age groups. They will diagnose and direct care for any congenital issue, such as hip dislocation, club feet, or any congenital malformation of the limbs. They are available to evaluate pronounced bowlegs, knock-knees, intoeing, outtoeing, strains, sprains, fractures, and scoliosis as your children grow.

Infectious Disease

The pediatric infectious disease subspecialist has a special interest in childhood infection. Infections are common in infancy and childhood, especially in the first two years of life, and most are viral, benign, and self-limited. Significant illness from infection can occur in children, which may prompt a consultation with this expert.

These subspecialists first complete the general pediatric training program, followed by a three-year fellowship in pediatric infectious disease. Usually active in clinical and academic medicine, they may be found in large teaching institutions and children's hospitals. They often divide their time between active research; teaching medical students, interns, and residents; and seeing patients like your children when needed. Your pediatrician may consult this physician if your child has a significant infection, a rare cause of infection, or an illness that has an unclear cause.

CONCLUSION

By now, it may be time to sing "Happy Birthday" to your baby boy or girl, and we have traveled this first year of wellness together. Soon he or she will be a walking, talking toddler! We hope that you have been helped and encouraged by this book, and that you have gained comfort and confidence with the knowledge that you have attained. You may wish to pass it on to a friend or loved one who is about to embark on the same family adventure!

You can be very proud of yourself for becoming the mother that your child wants and needs . . . never doubt yourself. Moms are right until proven otherwise. You have learned and grown together during this year, and this will never be lost on your little one . . . he or she will continue to thrive because of your loving care.

Your child will cherish you always.

APPENDIX A

Baby's Records

Tests Record

TEST	DATE	RESULT
Newborn screening	_____	_____
Tuberculin (PPD)	_____	_____
Hemoglobin or Hematocrit	_____	_____
Urinalysis	_____	_____
Lead	_____	_____
Cholesterol	_____	_____
Vision	_____	_____
Hearing	_____	_____
Other	_____	_____
Other	_____	_____
Other	_____	_____
Other	_____	_____
Other	_____	_____
Other	_____	_____

Record of Allergy or Sensitivity

DATE	AGE	ALLERGY/SENSITIVITY/REACTION

APPENDIX B

Important Contact Information

PEDIATRICIAN

Name _____

Address _____

Phone _____

Fax _____

E-mail _____

INSURANCE INFORMATION

Name _____

Address _____

Phone _____

Group No. _____

HOSPITAL

Address _____

Phone _____

PHARMACY

Address _____

Phone _____

POISON CONTROL CENTER

Phone _____

INDEX

Index

ABOUT THE AUTHOR

Dr. Peter Richel has been in practice for more than twenty years in suburban New York. He is on the teaching faculty at Albert Einstein College of Medicine and New York Medical College. He is now Chief of Pediatrics at Northern Westchester Hospital in Mount Kisco, New York. Along the way he co-produced a CD of his songs called "Dr. Pete's Office," with the hope of preventing children's fear of the doctor. He regularly appeared at Borders Books in Mount Kisco, singing for the children and speaking to them about health and wellness. He has appeared on *The Early Show* and *Eyewitness News* on ABC, CBS local and national news, and the national Sirius Radio show "On Call for Kids." He is often featured in local newspapers and magazines. A television show for preschool children is in the works. Please visit him at www.drpetesoffice.com.